The Tapestry of
MEMORY

Unraveling the Threads of the Mind

David L. Priede, PhD

The Tapestry of MEMORY: Unraveling the Threads of the Mind

Copyright © by David Priede, PhD

ISBN: 979-8-89379-801-2

The information included in this book is for educational purposes only. It is not intended or implied to be a substitute for professional medical advice. Readers should always consult a physician or healthcare provider to determine the appropriate information for their situation or questions regarding a medical condition or treatment plan. Reading the information in this book does not constitute a physician-patient relationship. The Food and Drug Administration (FDA) has not evaluated some of the book's statements. The author and publisher expressly disclaim responsibility for any adverse effects resulting from using or applying the information in this book.

Art design by Daló

Biolife Publishing
16175 Golf Club Road, Suite 108
Weston, FL 33326
10 9 8 7 6 5 4 3 2 1

Table of Contents

Dedication

To all the devoted scientists, researchers, and clinicians exploring the complexities of the human brain, your contributions are invaluable to our understanding of one of nature's most intricate creations. But let's also extend gratitude to people passionate about improving memory, cognition, and mental well-being. Your curiosity and pursuit of better memory techniques and cognitive enhancements make scientific advancements accessible and relevant.

Whether you are diligently practicing memory-enhancing exercises, spreading awareness about mental health, or advocating for more research, you play a critical role in broadening the impact of scientific findings. You bridge the gap between the laboratory and the living room, bringing practical applications into daily life.

Your involvement, no matter how small it may seem, also lights the path to a future where better understanding and management of our cognitive faculties is possible for everyone. Thank you for being part of this collective endeavor to unlock the full potential of the human brain.

About The Author

Dr. David L. Priede, PhD - Author

As a distinguished healthcare professional, Dr. David L. Priede has dedicated his career to propelling progress and fostering innovation. With a rich background in healthcare and technology, he has consistently challenged conventional boundaries and pioneered transformative solutions to address pressing challenges in these interconnected fields.

In the healthcare realm, Dr. Priede's dedication is unwavering. He has immersed himself in the intricacies of healthcare, striving to enhance patient care and outcomes by integrating cutting-edge technologies and evidence-based practices. His approach transcends traditional healthcare paradigms, embracing interdisciplinary collaboration and innovative methodologies.

At the forefront of technology, he has spearheaded initiatives leveraging emerging technologies to revolutionize healthcare delivery, improve operational efficiencies, and empower individuals to proactively manage their health. His work ranges from developing state-of-the-art medical devices to implementing data-driven solutions for predictive analytics and personalized medicine, consistently pushing boundaries at the intersection of technology and healthcare.

Furthermore, his commitment to research has been steadfast. He has dedicated countless hours to advancing scientific knowledge and driving forward the frontiers of medical discovery. Whether pioneering new therapies, unraveling disease mechanisms, or exploring innovative healthcare delivery approaches, Dr. Priede is driven by a relentless pursuit of excellence and a passion for contributing to the greater body of knowledge.

In addition to his professional achievements, he is a published science author, contributing to disseminating knowledge and furthering scientific understanding in his areas of expertise.

His academic journey reflects a dedication to education and research, with degrees ranging from Computer Science and Engineering to Medical Information Systems and Bioinformatics, culminating in a Ph.D. in Applied Sciences, further bolstering his science, technology, and research expertise.

Furthermore, his active involvement in esteemed professional organizations such as The American Medical Association, The National Association for Healthcare Quality, The Society for Neuroscience, and The American Brain Foundation keeps him abreast of the latest advancements and fosters collaboration with fellow experts in the field.

Other titles by Dr. David L. Priede
-The Conditions Afflicting the Body, Mind, and Soul of America
-The Future of Health: Emerging Technologies

Gabriella Chianese – Collaborator

A trailblazer in her own right, Gabriella Chianese graduated from the University of New Hampshire with dual degrees in Biomedical Sciences and Political Science, complemented by an accelerated master's in molecular and cellular biotechnology. Her academic journey was marked by an impressive track record of leadership, having served as the president of multiple student organizations, inspiring and guiding her peers with unwavering dedication.

Chianese's contributions extend far beyond the confines of the classroom, as she actively engaged in academic research, civic engagement, and volunteer work throughout her studies, showcasing her commitment to making a lasting positive impact.

As a recent graduate, Gabriella Chianese stands as an inspiration, having already left an indelible mark on the communities she served. With her remarkable academic achievements, leadership capabilities, and unwavering commitment to service, she is poised to make significant contributions to both the scientific and political realms, paving the way for a future filled with boundless potential.

Karis Bittner – Collaborator

Karis Bittner, a Forensic Anthropology graduate from Texas Tech University, has seamlessly blended her academic passion with a commitment to community service. Beyond her expertise in the field, Bittner has acquired a remarkable array of certifications, including lifeguard, nurse assistant, and EMT, underscoring her dedication to saving lives and providing compassionate care.

Bittner's altruistic spirit transcends her academic endeavors, as evidenced by her active involvement in various organizations. She has been a part of the Girl Scouts, fostering leadership and personal growth, and a member of the American Association of Biological Anthropologists, further deepening her understanding of her chosen field. Her volunteerism has taken her on a remarkable journey, from participating in Relay for Life to support cancer research and services, to embarking on mission work in the Dominican Republic, where she contributed her time and efforts to uplift the local community. Additionally, Bittner's dedication to cultural exchange led her to teach English in China, fostering cross-cultural understanding and enriching the lives of her students.

With her multifaceted skillset, academic excellence, and commitment to serving others, Bittner exemplifies the harmonious fusion of intellectual pursuit and humanitarian ideals, leaving a mark on the communities she has touched.

Lindsey Delacour – Senior Editor

Lindsey Delacour, armed with a degree in English Literature from Clarion University in Pennsylvania, brings a unique blend of creative spirit, technical prowess, artistic flair, and masterful storytelling to every endeavor she undertakes. With a keen eye for detail and an unwavering passion for language, she excels at crafting compelling narratives while ensuring unwavering accuracy and clarity.

Beyond her impressive editorial abilities, Delacour is driven by an insatiable desire to share her imaginative fiction stories with the world through the written word. She actively pursues publication opportunities, tirelessly refining her craft and pouring her heart into bringing her innovative narratives to life on the printed page.

A member of The Author's Guild, she is deeply embedded in the literary community, continuously honing her skills and seeking inspiration from fellow authors.

Delacour's artistic talents extend beyond the realm of words, as she has showcased her paintings contributing to the vibrant local artistic community. Her multifaceted creative spirit allows her to approach projects with a unique perspective, blending technical expertise with a deep appreciation for aesthetics and storytelling.

Lindsey Delacour is a true Renaissance individual, seamlessly blending artistic expression, literary prowess, and a deep appreciation for language and storytelling, leaving an indelible mark on every endeavor she pursues.

One weekend, I stumbled upon a charming bookstore and was captivated by a book with an eye-catching cover. I bought it, went home, and spent hours engrossed in its pages. The story was riveting, filled with complex characters and unexpected twists. That night, I closed the book, feeling fulfilled and nostalgic for the fictional world I had just left behind.

A few months later, a friend asked for a book recommendation. Unsurprisingly, I thought of that unforgettable read. But to my surprise, I could not recall the specifics—neither the main character nor the major plot points. It felt like a treasured experience had somehow slipped from my memory.

David L. Priede

April 3ᵗʰ, 2024

Introduction

We are all on a journey to become the best versions of ourselves, and achieving better health often tops our list. The good news is that advances in research offer us new and exciting ways to improve our lives. One of the most eye-opening discoveries focuses on how we can care for our memory.

While we've always heard that eating well and staying active is important, there's much more. For instance, recent studies suggest that certain mental practices can serve as a 'gym' for our brain, improving focus and cognitive agility.

Do you sometimes find yourself worried about forgetfulness? This book will help you understand how memory works and the factors affecting your brain's function and performance. You'll find actionable steps to boost and maintain your memory. You'll also discover a range of practical strategies for enhancing your everyday recollection.

Your brain is more than just a storage vault for memories; it's a dynamic and vibrant part of you that influences how you learn, interact with others, and tackle life's challenges. And let's not forget that emotional well-being also plays a pivotal role in cognitive health. While factors like aging, stress, and other health issues can affect memory, the uplifting news is that we're not helpless. We can take proactive steps to improve our brain's performance.

Longevity presents both opportunities and challenges when it comes to memory. On the bright side, living longer—*thanks in part to advances in healthcare*—means more chances to create and cherish beautiful memories. On the flip side, aging alters the way our brain functions. But let's focus on the positive: these changes don't have to be setbacks. It's important to remember that the brain's plasticity allows us to adapt and learn throughout our lives. In fact, with the right approach, we can slow or even counteract the effects of aging to maintain a robust memory.

In this book, you'll find an empowering guide to understand and take charge of your brain's health with tips and strategies to keep it agile and vibrant. This guide is more than just a handbook; it's a tool to maximize your cognitive capabilities. So, let's embark on this exciting journey of discovery together. Here's to a life filled with clarity, vibrant memories, and an ever-curious and youthful mind!

CHAPTER 1

The Importance of Memory

Memory is essential to human cognition, serving as the brain's mechanism for retaining and recalling information. It encompasses vast knowledge, experiences, and moments, from academic learning to cherished interactions with loved ones. Memory empowers us to store, preserve, and access this wealth of information, shaping various aspects of our lives.

Memory is a fundamental aspect of human cognition that plays a pivotal role in our daily lives. In its most basic terms, memory is the process of the brain retaining and retrieving information. This information can come from various moments and seasons in our lives, ranging from knowledge gained by reading or schooling to experiences shared with loved ones.

Our memory enables us to store, retain, and retrieve information, including experiences and events from our past. Memory allows us to learn from our skills, make decisions based on our knowledge, and communicate effectively with others. Memories impact our lives in countless ways. Several aspects of our lives, such as learning skills, communication, and emotions, are shaped by our memories.

Our memory provides us with many functional and realistic benefits. Acquiring new knowledge, skills, and experiences can enhance our problem-solving abilities and strengthen our reasoning skills. Having a good memory can lead to better academic and job performance. Suppose you excel in complex tasks like following multi-step instructions, playing musical instruments, or math. In that case, you likely have a strong working memory, contributing significantly to our brain's ability to handle these tasks.

The benefits of a strong memory extend into our personal lives. Successful and meaningful communication or social interaction depends upon our ability to remember people's names and faces. Memory is essential to having effective conversations.

Our memory allows us to form bonds and maintain social relationships while enabling us to access relevant information and experiences to express our opinions or ideas more effectively.

The core of our being is our memory, and it safeguards our most treasured moments. It reflects our past, from lessons in old books to a mother's touch. These memories guide and shape us, reminding us of past joys and sorrows and giving us wisdom. Memories provide depth to our identity and aid us practically, enhancing our intellect and problem-solving abilities.

They connect us to others and help us navigate life, ensuring we remember faces, names, and shared experiences, making each life interaction more prosperous and profound.

Memory and You

Our memories play a primary role in shaping who we are, how we function, and how we relate to others. The lessons we learn early in our development become ingrained into the fiber of our being through memory storage. These lessons can range from the cautious warnings of our parents, caretakers, and schoolteachers to the more challenging ones we experience through our mistakes.

Often unknowingly, these lessons and the countless others we learn along the way inform our daily decision-making processes. We shape who we are by mediating our memories, using the ability to unlock and apply them. We recall, interpret, and apply our past experiences in our routines, habits, sense of identity, problem-solving skills, emotions, and social connections.

Learning and Retaining Information

Memory enables us to learn and retain information, varying from basic knowledge like language and simple math skills to more complex concepts such as scientific theories and historical events. With the aid of memory, we can learn and retain new information, continuously developing new skills and expanding our knowledge base. Moreover, a well-functioning memory is the foundation for lifelong learning, allowing us to adapt and evolve in an ever-changing world.

When we learn something new, our brain forms connections between neurons that help encode and store the information in our memory. These connections, known as synapses, strengthen over time through a process called synaptic plasticity, making it easier for us to recall the information later.

For example, in language learning, memory is key for remembering new vocabulary words, grammar rules, and sentence structures. By storing this information in our memory, we can build upon our language skills, ultimately becoming proficient writers and speakers.

Decision-Making

Our decision-making process heavily relies on memory. It enables us to recall past experiences, detect patterns, and establish connections among disparate pieces of information. These recollections subsequently influence our future choices. Our brain has multiple decision-making systems, and memory interacts seamlessly with them.

When faced with decisions, weighing many factors, such as individual desires, available external data, and prior experiences, is essential. Take, for instance, the scenario of receiving a job offer. While the financial benefits might be tempting, the company's negative reputation for employee satisfaction will help you make a better decision. Previous negative experiences in similar situations might deter you from accepting the job.

Problem-Solving

When addressing brain-based problem-solving, we must recognize various challenges, from creative dilemmas to mathematical reasoning. Memory processing significantly influences our ability to solve these problems, depending on our working memory capacity.

This process has two main stages: understanding the problem (representation phase) and finding a solution (solution phase). For instance, when you see an uneven sidewalk, you quickly assess the potential risk in the representation phase and adjust your step to avoid tripping in the solution phase.

Sense of Identity

Our identities are deeply rooted in our memories. Memory influences our beliefs, values, goals, and how we relate to others. This relationship between memory and identity is interconnected—our memories define our self-view, and our identities affect how we remember certain events.

For example, remember childhood experiences where you might have been teased or criticized by loved ones. Such memories can impact self-worth and confidence. As these

4

recollections resurface in daily life, they can reinforce insecurities. Episodic memory is responsible for recalling specific events, situations, and experiences from one's past; hence, it is deeply linked to our sense of self.

Adaptation to New Situations

By recalling past experiences, memory enables us to adjust to new circumstances. The effectiveness of our working memory lies in quickly recalling these experiences. This is especially vital when we must act swiftly, as our ability to connect current situations to past events is indispensable for making split-second decisions.

When presented with a problem that requires adaptability, there are multiple things to consider. For example, when driving, you make countless quick decisions based on the behavior of other drivers on the road, the physical environment, and vehicle conditions. Prior experience dealing with these varying factors allows you to filter through your options when confronted with a problem to choose the safest option.

Emotional Well-Being

Our memories deeply tie into our emotional health. Simple sensations, like the scent of a familiar perfume or the sound of an ice cream truck, can instantly transport us back to specific moments, evoking strong emotions. For instance, the taste of strawberries might remind us of a childhood garden, or the feel of soft fleece could recall a cherished blanket from our youth.

These sensory triggers interact with our autobiographical memory, grounding us in our personal histories and providing comfort through recognizing past joys. As we connect with these memories, we further solidify our identities, drawing from experiences that make us feel rooted and at home. On the flip side, certain stimuli can also bring up unpleasant memories. While such recollections can be unsettling, confronting and processing them can enhance our resilience and emotional growth.

Social Connections

Our memories interface with our connectivity to others and fuel social engagement. Consider all the factors that foster a solid foundation for your interpersonal relationships – you take solace in knowing that your friend remembers your birthday, your favorite ice cream flavor, the names of your parents or kids and that you hate pineapple on pizza.

The strength of your relationship relies on the information you remember about each other and your shared experiences. Our memories foster longevity and connectivity in our interpersonal relationships, but social connections also help improve memory. Additionally, social interaction primes our memory to safeguard against mental degradation and enhance cognition.

Maintaining regular, meaningful social connections throughout life provides cognitive stimulation, which may protect against cognitive decline later in life. Therefore, robust friendships and a vibrant social life may be an underappreciated defense against mental deterioration.

Reflections on The Importance of Memory

Memory is the foundation of our personal histories, allowing us to reminisce about past experiences and draw upon learned knowledge in present and future situations. It is the repository of our lives, a rich tapestry of events, emotions, and information, weaving together the intricate threads of our identities and relationships. Through memory, we forge connections between our past, present, and future, enabling us to navigate the complexities of life with a sense of continuity, coherence, and growth.

The ability to store and retrieve experiences is at the core of our memory. This capability is fundamental to our cognitive functions, including learning, decision-making, and problem-solving. By recalling past experiences and applying their lessons, we enhance our ability to adapt to new situations and challenges. This capacity for learning and adaptation is a cornerstone of human survival and progress, enabling us to acquire new skills, knowledge, and insights throughout our lives.

Memory also plays a critical role in shaping our personal narratives. It gives us a sense of identity and continuity, connecting us to our histories and cultural heritage. By understanding the significance of memory, we gain insights into the intricate tapestry of experiences and knowledge that shapes who we are and how we engage with the world.

CHAPTER 2

The Journey of Memory Creation

Our minds work daily as our senses gather data from the world around us. For instance, when you enter a coffee shop, your senses are engaged by the aroma of coffee, your eyes dart toward the menu, and your hands anticipate the warmth of a cozy cup. Memory involves stages imperative for absorbing, storing, and recalling this kind of information from our experiences.

O ur minds are capable of incredible feats. Each day, as we interact with the world around us, our bodies gather data from our environment through our five senses: sight, touch, sound, taste, and smell. These senses allow us to comprehend our surroundings. Consider walking into a coffee shop. The first thing that shapes your perception of the space is the aroma of freshly brewed coffee. Next, you glance at the menu, spotting favorites: a French vanilla latte and a chocolate croissant.

You place your order and patiently wait for the barista to call your name. Taking the to-go cup from the bar top, you feel the warmth between your hands before sipping your coffee. How long will you remember this experience, and which details will linger? What determines which specifics become encoded in our memory for us to reminisce about long after the moment, while others vanish like the fleeting coffee aroma?

The memory process can be divided into three stages: acquisition, consolidation, and retrieval. These three stages must seamlessly interact for complete memory processing to occur. Failure or delay at any of these memory processing levels can significantly impact our ability to absorb new information from the environment, store it for later use, and retrieve it when necessary.

Stage 1: Acquisition

Memory acquisition is not just a building block but the cornerstone of human cognition. This subject has piqued the curiosity of disciplines ranging from psychology and neuroscience to education and philosophy. This phase is where the raw data of our experiences—what we see, hear, smell, taste, and touch—get encoded into a language that our brains can understand and utilize. The initial step in a multi-stage journey includes consolidation and retrieval, enabling us to learn, make decisions, and interact with our environment.

This vital stage is the entry point for all our learning experiences and cognitive functions. It acts as a funnel, collecting a wide array of stimuli and then channeling them into our cognitive system. The process itself can be automatic or intentional, passive or active. Still, its role as the gatekeeper to our mind's intricate network is constant.

From the very first moments of life, when a newborn hears words and starts the incredible journey of language acquisition, all the way to the specialized skills honed by professionals over years of practice, memory acquisition is where it all begins. This phase allows a musician to remember scales, a student to memorize equations, or a traveler to recall the landmarks that guided them through unfamiliar terrain.

Moreover, memory acquisition is deeply interwoven with our emotional experiences and personal growth. Whether it's the pain or joy from life-changing events, these experiences first enter our cognitive system through acquisition. It helps shape our perspectives, attitudes, and future decisions.

Thus, memory acquisition is not merely a mechanical act but a dynamic process intertwined with our identities, goals, and essence. It shapes how we navigate complexities, solve problems, and form relationships. By understanding its nuances, we unlock the potential to enhance our cognitive abilities and gain a more profound understanding of the human experience.

Examples of Memory Acquisition

Memory acquisition is the initial stage of the memory process, where sensory input is collected from the environment and transformed into information that can be stored and retrieved later. Here are some examples of memory acquisition at work in everyday situations:

- *Classroom Learning:* Students acquire memory when listening to a teacher's lecture, taking notes, or participating in class discussions. They gather information from the teacher's words, visual aids, and peer interactions to retain that knowledge for exams and assignments.

- ***Reading a Book:*** When you read a book, your brain acquires information from the text. You absorb details about the plot, characters, and settings, temporarily stored in your short-term memory. As the story progresses, your brain consolidates essential information for long-term retention.
- ***Cooking a New Recipe:*** Trying a new recipe involves memory acquisition. You read the recipe, process the steps, and remember the ingredients and cooking techniques. This information is necessary to execute the recipe successfully and potentially remember it for future use.
- ***Navigating a New City:*** When you visit a new city and explore its streets, you acquire spatial and navigational information. Your brain processes landmarks, street names, and directions, helping you find your way around. This acquired knowledge may become useful if you revisit the city.
- ***Learning a Musical Instrument:*** Playing a musical instrument requires memory acquisition of musical notes, chords, and finger placements. Musicians acquire and memorize this information to play music. With practice, this knowledge becomes ingrained in long-term memory.
- ***Meeting New People:*** When meeting new people, you acquire information about their names, faces, and personal details. Your brain processes this information, and with repetition and interaction, you aim to consolidate it into long-term memory to remember these individuals in the future.
- ***Learning a New Language:*** Acquiring a new language involves memory acquisition of vocabulary, grammar rules, and pronunciation. Language learners repeatedly encounter new words and phrases in various contexts to facilitate memory consolidation.
- ***Watching a Documentary:*** You acquire information about a specific topic while watching a documentary or educational program. Your brain processes facts, statistics, and visual content to retain this knowledge for future discussions or applications.
- ***Participating in Work Training:*** Employees acquire new information related to their jobs during workplace training sessions or seminars. They learn about company policies, procedures, software tools, or industry-specific

knowledge to apply this acquired information in their work roles.

These examples demonstrate how memory acquisition plays a fundamental role in our daily lives, allowing us to gather information from our surroundings and experiences for immediate and long-term purposes.

Selective Encoding

The world around you bombard our senses with many stimuli, from sights and sounds to tastes and textures. Yet, encoding everything you encounter would quickly lead to cognitive overload, leaving little mental capacity for essential tasks like mental calculations, remembering a shopping list, or engaging in meaningful conversations with friends. It involves filtering incoming information to determine what is important and worthy of attention.

To navigate this information-rich environment, your brain employs selective encoding. This process filters and prioritizes sensory data for storage based on its perceived relevance. Selective encoding is evident in various contexts, such as learning, problem-solving, and memory tasks. Motivation can influence selective encoding, leading individuals to focus on information relevant to their goals.

Automatic Acquisition

Acquisition happens automatically as you interact with your surroundings, but it's not a passive process. Your attention, motivation, and the nature of the information you're processing are pivotal in determining what gets encoded. Research indicates that external stimuli linked to fear or strong emotions are more likely to be etched into your memory than those that elicit minimal emotional responses.

Information that holds personal relevance or carries emotional significance, such as a fear-inducing event or a heartwarming memory, tends to find its way into your long-term memory. Furthermore, this emotional component not only enhances the encoding process but also influences the retrieval and consolidation of memories, ensuring that these emotionally significant experiences remain readily accessible and enduring over time.

This emotional modulation of memory has important implications for various domains, including education, psychotherapy, and eyewitness testimony, where understanding the interplay between emotion and memory can inform more effective strategies for learning, processing traumatic experiences, and accurately recounting events.

The Extraordinary and the Mundane

Similarly, unique or exciting information stands a better chance of being encoded and later recalled. Consider your daily commute— a routine often so automated that you feel like you're on autopilot. If someone were to ask about your drive to work, you might briefly mention traffic conditions, the weather, or the music you listened to.

However, these minor details rarely make a lasting impression in your long-term memory. In contrast, more extraordinary or emotionally charged experiences readily take root in your memory, eclipsing the mundane details.

Stage 2: Consolidation

The consolidation process is the unsung hero of memory. It is often overshadowed by the more apparent acts of encoding and retrieval. Yet, it plays a pivotal role in shaping the memories that will stick with us throughout our lives.

After new information has been encoded, the consolidation process begins, acting as the forge that transforms these initial sparks of memory into enduring flames. This alchemical transformation enables you to recall essential facts, experiences, and knowledge even years after the original event.

Once the information is encoded, it doesn't stay in one single, isolated part of the brain. Instead, it's distributed and stored in various regions, depending on the memory type being processed— semantic, episodic, or procedural. This transition from initial stimulus processing to information storage is not just a data transfer but an essential refining process that solidifies the new memories and prepares them for long-term storage.

If you've ever delved into study strategies to improve your academic performance, you were looking for ways to make this memory processing more efficient. From spaced repetition techniques to mnemonics, various methods aim to aid the consolidation process to turn fleeting information into long-lasting knowledge.

However, it's essential to recognize that more than simple exposure to information is often required for effective consolidation. Listening to a lecture or scanning your notes might feel productive. Still, these efforts may not sufficiently trigger the consolidation process without engaging more deeply with the material—perhaps through active recall, elaboration, or contextual application.

Therefore, genuinely effective learning strategies involve a conscious effort to engage with the material on a deeper level, activating multiple cognitive and sensory pathways to solidify the information in our memory systems.

So, while you may initially engage with educational content and interact with environmental stimuli, these actions represent just the beginning of the intricate process of memory formation. The true magic frequently occurs backstage, during the critical yet often underappreciated consolidation phase.

This essential phase involves a series of complex neural processes that work in synergy to strengthen the connections between different brain regions, leading to the successful storage and recall of memories. Although it may not always be obvious or readily apparent, the consolidation phase plays a key role in the intricate tapestry of memory creation and retrieval.

Examples of Memory Consolidation

Memory consolidation is the process by which newly acquired information or skills are stabilized and integrated into your existing knowledge base, making them easier to access and utilize later. Here are some examples that illustrate this concept.

- ***Studying for an Exam:*** When you first read through your study materials, the information is fresh and may require frequent review. As you revisit the material and perhaps even sleep on it, your brain works to make this information more stable and more accessible to recall when needed.
- ***Learning to Ride a Bike:*** Balancing and pedaling may require much focus and conscious effort. However, with repeated practice and some rest, your brain integrates this skill into your existing abilities, making it almost automatic.
- ***Cooking a New Recipe:*** First, you may need to continually refer to the recipe for each step and ingredient. Over time and with repeated cooking, your brain stabilizes this information, allowing you to prepare the dish without constantly checking the instructions.
- ***Musical Practice:*** When learning a new piece of music, you may have to look at sheet music frequently. With

enough repetition, your brain integrates the notes and rhythms, enabling you to repeatedly perform without referring to the written music.

- **Language Learning:** Newly learned vocabulary and grammatical rules may initially require active thought and effort. However, these elements become more integrated and easier to use in conversation and comprehension through exposure and practice.
- **Emotional Events:** Strong emotional experiences often become deeply integrated into your memory due to the involvement of emotional centers in the brain. For example, the amygdala is a part of the limbic system. It is primarily associated with emotional processing, including fear, anxiety, and aggression.
- **Spatial Navigation:** When you first move to a new place, you may rely heavily on maps and GPS. As you become more familiar with the area, your brain makes this spatial information more stable, allowing you to navigate without assistance.
- **Professional Skills:** In any job, there are specific skills and knowledge that you must acquire. This information becomes more integrated through training and hands-on experience, helping you perform your job more efficiently.
- **Childhood Learning:** Basic life skills like walking and talking are initially challenging but become more integrated into your skill set as you grow, to the point where you can perform them without conscious thought.
- **Medical Procedures:** Learning procedures and protocols are Important for healthcare professionals. Repeated practice and application make these more stable and easier to perform, leading to more effective patient care.

In each of these examples, memory consolidation helps to make newly acquired information or skills more stable and accessible when needed.

Stage 3: Retrieval

Memory retrieval is a critical mechanism in the functioning of the human mind. It enables us to access and bring forth information that has been previously encoded and stored within our neural networks. Far from being a simple replay, memory retrieval is a dynamic and intricate process that mobilizes various cognitive and neural resources. It engages multiple brain regions and pathways, underscoring its complexity and centrality to human cognition.

Memory retrieval is not just a background function but fundamental to a range of cognitive functions central to our daily lives.

For example, problem-solving is not just about innate intelligence or creativity; it often hinges on our ability to retrieve and apply principles or facts we have previously learned. This capability enables us to tackle new challenges by applying tried-and-true methods or adapting past solutions to fit new scenarios.

Similarly, effective decision-making is deeply rooted in our memory functions. Whether deciding on a career path or choosing what to eat for dinner, our decisions are informed by our ability to recall past experiences, weigh outcomes, and even remember the judgments we or others have made. This retrieval process adds depth and sophistication to our decision-making, allowing us to make informed and nuanced choices.

Social interactions, too, are heavily dependent on memory retrieval. Our ability to navigate social environments—be it a family gathering, a workplace setting, or even an online community—is facilitated by our memory systems. Recognizing faces, recalling names, and even remembering important dates or social norms and cues are all made possible by the complex memory retrieval process. Without this capability, every social encounter would be confusing, lacking context or history.

Thus, memory retrieval is not merely a function of the mind but a cornerstone of our cognitive architecture. It profoundly influences various aspects of our lives, from the intellectual to the emotional and social, shaping our experiences and interactions.

Stages of Memory Retrieval

1. *Cue-Dependent Retrieval:* The first step in retrieving a memory often involves a cue or trigger. This could be a word, an image, a smell, or even a feeling associated with the memory you're trying to recall. For example, the scent of freshly baked cookies triggers memories of your grandmother's kitchen.

2. *Search and Activation:* Once a cue is presented, your brain begins to search for its stored information. Neural pathways that were formed when the memory was encoded are activated. This is often a rapid process but can vary in speed and accuracy depending on various factors like the

age of the memory, emotional intensity, or how often it has been recalled before.

3. **Reconstruction:** Human memory is reconstructive, unlike a computer, which stores data in a fixed format. This means that remembering often involves piecing together various components of the stored information. Sometimes, this can lead to inaccuracies or distortions in the recalled memory.

4. **Conscious Awareness:** After the memory has been located and reconstructed, it surfaces into your conscious awareness, enabling you to engage with it actively, share it with others, or contemplate its significance at leisure.

5. **Reconsolidation:** After a memory has been retrieved, it often undergoes a process of reconsolidation, where it is re-stored with any new information or context that may have been added during the retrieval process. This can sometimes alter the original memory.

Examples of Memory Retrieval

Memory retrieval is a complex cognitive function that allows us to access and utilize information that has been previously encoded and stored. This process is crucial for a wide range of activities and scenarios. Here are some examples to illustrate the concept:

- **Recognizing a Face:** When you run into someone you've met before, your brain quickly retrieves the stored information about that person, allowing you to recognize them and perhaps even recall their name and other details about your past interactions.
- **Taking a Test:** During an exam, you retrieve various pieces of information you've learned, whether historical dates, mathematical formulas, or literary themes, to answer questions effectively.
- **Driving a Car:** When you drive, you're constantly retrieving learned skills and rules—like when to brake, how to make a turn, or what a particular road sign means—without even realizing it.
- **Telling a Story:** When you share an anecdote or recount an event, you're engaging in memory retrieval. You recall the main events and details like who was there, what was said, and how you felt.
- **Navigating Your Hometown:** If you've lived in the same place for many years, you can probably get around

without a map or GPS. This involves retrieving spatial memories of streets, landmarks, and routes.

- ***Playing a Musical Instrument:*** Skilled musicians can play songs from memory, retrieving not just the notes but also the nuances of tempo, volume, and emotion that go into a performance.
- ***Responding to Smells or Sounds:*** Certain smells or sounds can instantly trigger vivid memories. For example, the scent of a specific perfume might remind you of a particular person, or the sound of a song might take you back to a specific time and place.
- ***Speaking a Second Language:*** If you're bilingual or multilingual, you retrieve vocabulary and grammatical rules of the language you're using, often switching between languages seamlessly.
- ***Shopping:*** At the grocery store, you retrieve a mental list of items you need, even if you haven't written them down. You might also recall which aisles contain the products you're looking for.
- ***Emergency Situations:*** In urgent scenarios, like a fire or medical emergency, you retrieve Important information on how to respond, such as stopping, dropping, and rolling if your clothes catch fire or performing CPR on someone unconscious.

Memory retrieval is imperative for informed decision-making, problem-solving, and social interactions. It allows us to access stored information and apply past experiences and knowledge to current situations. This complex cognitive function is essential for navigating our daily lives effectively. Moreover, memory retrieval plays a critical role in shaping our identities, as recalling past experiences and emotions contributes to forming our self-concept, perceptions, and overall sense of self.

Brain Areas Involved in Acquisition, Consolidation, and Retrieval

Memory is a complex and multifaceted process that can be examined at various levels, from the macroscopic scale of behavior to the microscopic scale of individual neurons. Exploring memory at both the psychological and neural levels is essential to appreciate its intricacies fully.

At the psychological level, memory is often divided into three stages: acquisition, consolidation, and retrieval. Each of these stages involves specific brain regions that work together in a coordinated manner to create, store, and retrieve memories. By gaining insights into the roles of different brain regions in memory processes, researchers and educators can develop more effective strategies for enhancing memory performance, improving learning and academic achievement, and addressing memory-related disorders.

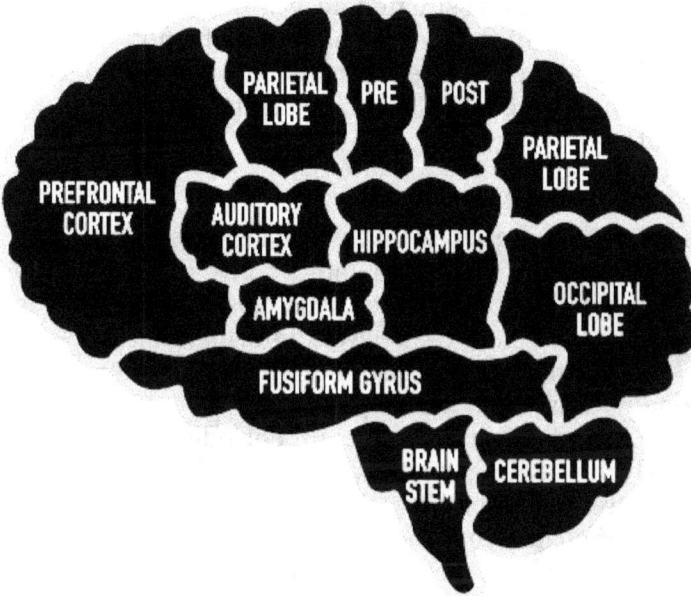

Figure 1

Memory Acquisition

The **hippocampus** is located in the **medial temporal lobe** and is essential for encoding new memories. It helps associate different types of information from various sensory channels and plays a role in spatial memory. Another critical area is the **prefrontal cortex**, particularly vital for working memory, which temporarily holds information for immediate use. This region allows for the manipulation of information. It is involved in decision-making processes that could influence what gets stored in long-term memory.

Memory Consolidation

The **hippocampus** is again involved in this process, but the shift of responsibility gradually moves toward the **neocortex**. The neocortex is the outer layer of the cerebral hemispheres. It is implicated in higher-order brain functions such as perception, reasoning, and decision-making. Research indicates that during sleep, the hippocampus and neocortex communicate to strengthen the neural connections that form memories, effectively "transferring" them for long-term storage.

Another area worth mentioning is the **amygdala**, an almond-shaped cluster of nuclei situated deep within the temporal lobe. It is especially relevant for the consolidation of emotional memories. Emotional experiences often become deeply engrained, thanks partly to the amygdala's role in tagging these memories as significant.

Memory Retrieval

The **prefrontal cortex** takes on a key role again. This area is involved in recalling memories and is active when individuals are asked to remember past events. It is closely associated with the hippocampus to pull out the relevant information.

The **parietal lobe** is also noteworthy. Although it is not traditionally considered a core part of the memory system, recent research suggests it has a role in episodic memory retrieval, particularly in orienting the individual to the spatial and contextual aspects of a recalled memory.

The **cerebellum and basal ganglia** are two other regions involved in procedural memory, responsible for skills like riding a bike or playing an instrument. These areas are not engaged in the conscious recall of memories. Still, they are indispensable for tasks that have become automatic through repetition.

Reflections on The Journey of Memory Creation

The interplay between mental and emotional states and memory retention is a fascinating aspect of human cognition. Our ability to remember information is not merely a matter of repetition. It is significantly influenced by our level of engagement, emotional connection, and contextual factors. Exploring this intricate relationship can provide valuable insights for enhancing memory function and optimizing cognitive performance.

18

When we are deeply engaged in a subject or activity, our brains are more likely to encode and retain that information. This phenomenon is often observed in educational settings, where active learning and participation are encouraged to foster better understanding and memory retention. By tapping into this natural propensity of the brain, educators can design more effective teaching methods that engage students and enhance their learning experiences.

Emotional significance also plays a critical role in shaping our memories. Emotionally charged events, whether joyous or traumatic, tend to leave a lasting imprint on our memory. This phenomenon can be attributed to the release of stress hormones during emotional experiences, heightening alertness and attention, leading to more vivid and persistent memories. Understanding this connection between emotion and memory can help us navigate our personal experiences and relationships more effectively.

It is important to note that memory is not just a passive repository of information; it is an active and dynamic process that is intimately linked with our emotional state, social interactions, and contextual settings. Recognizing the complexities of human memory and the factors that influence it can empower us to devise strategies for improving memory function, whether for academic or professional success or for enhancing our personal lives and relationships.

In conclusion, the intricate relationship between memory and our mental and emotional conditions is a captivating aspect of human cognition. Exploring this interplay can provide valuable insights for optimizing memory function and enhancing our overall cognitive performance. By understanding the impact of engagement, emotional significance, and contextual factors on memory, we can devise strategies to support learning, navigate personal experiences, and ultimately enrich our lives and relationships.

CHAPTER 3

Types of Memory

Memory is a remarkable tapestry woven from our experiences, emotions, and cognition. It's a record of life's events and a powerful influencer on our decisions, identities, and perceptions. Our memory is selective, prioritizing what's most significant to us, whether recalling the details of a past adventure or the scent of a childhood aroma.

Have you ever found yourself lost in thought, marveling at how precisely you can recount the nuances of an old hiking adventure—the fresh scent of pine trees, the distant chirping of birds, and the breathtaking landscapes—yet draw a blank when trying to recall what you had for dinner just yesterday?

Memory is not merely a repository for life's moments; it's a complex tapestry intricately woven from the threads of experience, raw emotion, and keen cognition. This tapestry doesn't just catalog events; it profoundly influences our decisions, shapes our identities, and colors our perceptions of the world.

Consider those moments when a familiar aroma from childhood momentarily stops you in your tracks or how, after years, you can still flawlessly execute the steps of a dance you once mastered. Our memory process isn't uniform. In fact, it's tailored and ranked based on what our conscious minds deem most significant or impactful. As we delve deeper into this topic, we will uncover the layers and mechanisms constituting memory, illuminating its diverse types, vital functions, and sophisticated processes at its core.

Memory Types

Memory serves as the mind's library, cataloging experiences and knowledge that shape our understanding of the world and ourselves. However, memory isn't just a singular, unified function. It's a multifaceted system with various types, each playing a distinct role in recalling, processing, and storing information.

From the immediate impressions that barely last a second to deeply ingrained recollections from years past, different types of memory engage to ensure we function effectively in our daily lives. In this exploration, we will navigate the diverse landscape of memory types and shed light on the mechanisms behind each.

Memory falls into the following four primary categories: sensory, short-term, working memory, and long-term.

Sensory Memory

Have you ever reminisced about relaxing on a beach? Reflecting on this memory, you can almost recall the sensations: the salty aroma of the ocean, the feel of the sand beneath your feet, and the vast horizon of waves. Such vivid recollections are courtesy of your sensory memory.

Sensory memory captures the immediate sensations from our environment. It allows us to momentarily retain experiences related to sight, taste, touch, and smell. Though fleeting, typically lasting less than a second, sensory memory plays an important role in shaping our more extended memory. It encompasses three primary registers: echoic, iconic, and haptic, each holding data briefly and fading quickly.

1. ***Echoic Memory:*** Echoic memory pertains to auditory retention, which is vital for processing language. Instead of only recognizing sounds, echoic memory helps us derive meaning from spoken words, enabling comprehension beyond mere listening. Iconic memory deals with visuals.

2. ***Iconic Memory:*** We tap into iconic memory when we conjure an image after its absence. This register has a significant capacity but is short-lived. There's an ongoing debate about its degradation. While some believe it fades gradually like an aging photograph, others argue it disappears rapidly.

3. ***Haptic or Tactile Memory:*** This type is rooted in touch. It lingers slightly longer than its counterparts, approximately 2 seconds. Although brief, once a tactile experience registers, it's more readily committed to long-term memory.

Short-term Memory

Short-term memory, also known as working memory, temporarily stores processed information. This type of memory lets us retain a small amount of information for a brief duration, typically less than 30 seconds. Short-term memory is pivotal in human cognition, enabling us to manipulate data, make choices, and tackle problems.

Individuals have varying capacities for short-term memory. Most people can hold around seven items, plus or minus two, in their short-term memory. Yet, using chunking techniques, we can enhance this capacity. Instead of trying to remember a disjointed series of letters like "DENFNLK," we can group them into recognizable chunks such as "DEN," "FNL," and "K."

Several factors, including distractions, can hinder short-term memory, making it challenging to retain and process information. Stress and anxiety can also negatively affect our ability to concentrate and, consequently, our short-term memory.

A robust short-term memory is vital for daily reading, listening, and problem-solving activities. It provides a temporary storage space for information, assisting us in decision-making and problem-solving. Understanding how short-term memory functions and using strategies like chunking and repetition can enhance cognitive performance in daily tasks.

Working Memory

Working memory is a dynamic and essential component of human cognition, often described as a mental "workspace." It temporarily stores and manipulates information, allowing us to perform various tasks that require storage and processing. Unlike other types of memory that hold information for later retrieval, working memory is unique in its ability to let us work with this information in real time.

This makes it indispensable for a wide range of various cognitive activities, such as solving complex mathematical problems, understanding language, learning new skills, and navigating unfamiliar environments.

Components of Working Memory

The most widely accepted model of working memory is the Baddeley-Hitch model, which proposes that working memory consists of three main components:

1. ***Central Executive:*** This control system directs attention to and processes activities. It decides what information is relevant and what should be ignored.

2. ***Phonological Loop:*** This component is responsible for holding verbal and auditory information. It's like a mental notepad where you rehearse phone numbers or directions.
3. ***Visuospatial Sketchpad:*** This is where visual and spatial information is processed. For example, it helps you remember a room's layout or a face's features.

Working memory is a dynamic and essential facet of human cognition. It serves as a temporary storage system that holds information and allows for its manipulation. This makes it important for various cognitive tasks, from problem-solving and decision-making to learning and social interaction.

Understanding the intricacies of working memory enriches our grasp of human cognition. It has practical implications in education, healthcare, and daily life.

Long-term Memory

Recalling the name of a family member or close friend seems almost instinctual, so deeply embedded that it's hard to imagine ever forgetting. Such enduring memories, which mold our lives and define our identities, reside in our long-term memory.

This system provides the most extended duration of storage, capturing a vast array of experiences and knowledge that shape who we are. Long-term memory is the longest-lasting storage available to us.

Long-term memory serves as an essential foundation of human cognition. However, it's not just a singular, monolithic system but a constellation of diverse subtypes, each uniquely designed to store and retrieve varying forms of information. Here's a detailed exploration of these primary long-term memory categories (explicit and implicit):

Explicit (or Declarative) Memory

This type of memory encompasses information we consciously think about and can verbally describe. Most people refer to it when they use the term "memory." Explicit memory is vital in our daily lives, as it helps us recall events, facts, figures, and locations. It's the form of memory you utilize when studying for an exam, telling a friend about your weekend, or recounting the plot of a movie.

Explicit memory is further classified into two main subcategories:

1. **Episodic Memory:** Episodic memory involves the capacity to retrieve precise events and experiences from our personal history, akin to viewing snapshots of those moments. These memories are uniquely individual, marked by timestamps, and rich in sensory details and emotions. Consider the sensations felt during a surprise birthday party or the sights and sounds etched in your memory from a remarkable vacation. Episodic memory stores these distinct occurrences and their intricate particulars, such as the gentle touch of the beach breeze during a holiday or the taste of the cake on your most recent birthday.

2. **Semantic Memory:** is our mental repository for general world knowledge unrelated to personal experience. It includes facts, concepts, and ideas. If you know the capital of a country you've never visited, understand the basic principles of mathematics, or recognize the meaning of a word you haven't personally encountered in a narrative, you're utilizing semantic memory. For instance, you might know a triangle has three sides but can't recall when or where you learned that fact. That's semantic memory in action.

Implicit (or Procedural) Memory

This type of memory involves memories that become almost automatic through repetition and do not require conscious thought. Procedural memory pertains to actions and skills, such as effortlessly playing a familiar song on the piano after years of practice.

Priming, a form of implicit memory, occurs when exposure to one stimulus unconsciously influences the response to another. For example, if you were previously shown the word "beach" and then asked to complete the word "s_nd," you might quickly respond with "sand" due to the prior association.

Implicit memory encompasses various forms of memory that operate without conscious awareness or intentional retrieval. There are indeed five primary types of implicit memory:

1. **Procedural Memory:** This type of memory involves recalling skills and procedures, such as riding a bike, typing on a keyboard, or playing a musical instrument. It is often characterized by the ability to perform tasks automatically after sufficient practice.

2. **Associative Memory:** Associative memory involves forming connections between related concepts or items. For example, if you associate the word "apple" with "fruit," this

linkage is stored implicitly. When you think of one, it may automatically trigger thoughts of the other.

3. **Non-Associative Memory:** Non-associative memory recognizes and responds to single stimuli without forming associations. Habituation and sensitization are common examples. Habituation is when a response to a repeated stimulation diminishes over time (e.g., tuning out background noise), while sensitization is an increased response to an intense or novel stimulus (e.g., jumping at a sudden loud noise).

4. **Priming:** Priming is a form of implicit memory where exposure to one stimulus influences the response to a related stimulus. For instance, if you see the word "yellow," you might recognize "banana" more quickly in a subsequent word association task.

5. **Perceptual Memory:** This type of memory relates to the recognition and identification of previously encountered sensory stimuli, such as faces, objects, or sounds. It allows us to recognize familiar faces or distinguish between sounds based on past experiences.

Implicit memory operates in the background, influencing our actions, thoughts, and perceptions without us consciously realizing it. Implicit memory collectively contributes to our ability to navigate and interact with the world efficiently.

Implicit memory operates outside of conscious awareness, and individuals may not realize how much it influences their daily actions and behaviors. It contrasts with explicit memory, where information can be consciously retrieved and articulated. Together, implicit and explicit memory systems contribute to our overall memory capabilities.

Emotional (Affective) Memory

Emotional Memory, also known as Affective Memory, is an essential aspect of our memory system that focuses on retaining and recalling emotions and associated experiences. Unlike factual or semantic memory, which stores objective information, emotional memory centers around the subjective and often visceral feelings tied to past events. It involves storing and retrieving emotional responses, such as joy, fear, sadness, or excitement, connected to specific experiences or situations.

This type of memory is particularly effective because it can significantly impact our decision-making, behavior, and overall well-being. Various stimuli, such as sights, sounds, or scents, can trigger emotional memories. They can evoke intense emotional reactions when recalled.

Emotional memory encompasses a spectrum of experiences that leave lasting imprints on our emotions and behaviors. Your first love, with its intense emotions of joy or heartache, remains etched in emotional memory years later. Traumatic events, like accidents or natural disasters, create enduring emotional imprints, potentially leading to post-traumatic stress disorder (PTSD). Positive and negative Childhood memories, such as birthday parties, continue to evoke nostalgia or emotional weight.

Personal achievements, such as winning a sports competition or earning an academic award, negatively impact our emotional memory. These memories are powerful motivators, boosting our self-esteem and driving us to pursue further successes. They also provide a source of resilience during challenging times, reminding us of our capabilities and encouraging us to persevere.

On the other hand, emotional memories associated with loss and grief also have a profound impact on our lives. Losing a loved one generates bittersweet memories that connect us to their memory, often evoking a mix of sadness and gratitude for the time we shared with them. These emotional memories can shape our perspectives on life and death, influencing our attitudes and behaviors in significant ways.

Moreover, emotional memories play an important role in the development of phobias and fears. For instance, a traumatic childhood encounter with a dog can lead to a lasting fear of dogs, influencing an individual's behavior and choices throughout their life. Similarly, past experiences of anxiety during public speaking can become imprinted in our emotional memory, impacting our future willingness to engage in similar situations.

Interestingly, sensory experiences, such as hearing a particular song, smelling a specific scent, or visiting a familiar place, can trigger emotional memories, transporting us back to a particular time and place in our lives. These sensory-emotional connections are often surprisingly powerful and vivid, evoking a wide range of emotions and associations.

In essence, emotional memories, whether positive or negative, shape our experiences, attitudes, and behaviors in significant ways. They serve as a connection to our past, influencing our present and future and contributing to the richness and complexity of our emotional lives. Understanding and managing emotional memories is key for emotional well-being and personal growth, as it allows individuals to harness the power of these memories for positive outcomes while mitigating their adverse effects.

Flashbulb Memory: A Unique Cognitive Phenomenon

Flashbulb memory occupies a particular niche within cognitive psychology, distinguished by its vividness and the emotional resonance of the events it captures. These memories of significant and often unexpected events remain etched in our minds in striking detail.

Vividness and Detail

One of the defining characteristics of flashbulb memories is their incredible clarity. Individuals can recall the main event and its peripheral details—where they were, what they were doing, and even what they wore when the event occurred.

Emotional Charge and Shared Experience

These memories often revolve around events carrying a significant emotional weight, personal or societal. Such emotional intensity aids in firmly embedding the memory. Often, these memories are formed in response to major societal events, leading to shared collective experiences. For instance, events like the 9/11 terrorist attacks or the news of Princess Diana's death have left indelible flashbulb memories in many minds.

Consistency and Confidence

Despite the natural tendency for memories to decay or distort over time, flashbulb memories remain remarkably consistent in their core elements. Individuals are typically confident about their recollection's accuracy, even if minute details vary upon close examination.

Biological Basis

From a neuroscientific perspective, the intense emotional reactions associated with such memories might lead to the release of stress hormones, enhancing memory consolidation. While flashbulb memories stand out for their clarity and emotional depth, they, like all memories, can be subject to change over time. Their vividness does not necessarily guarantee absolute accuracy. Still, it does underscore the profound impact certain events can have on our cognitive landscape.

Reflections on Types of Memory

Memory, in all its complexity and beauty, is the very essence of our existence. It is the intricate web that connects our past, present, and future, enabling us to learn, grow, and evolve as individuals. Just as a skilled artisan weaves a tapestry, so too does our memory weave together the vibrant threads of our experiences, emotions, and thoughts, creating a rich and multifaceted representation of our lives.

At the heart of this tapestry lies the remarkable diversity of memory types. From the instantaneous imprints of sensory memory to the enduring impressions of long-term memory, each layer contributes to the intricate mosaic of our identities. Whether it's the scent of a loved one's perfume, the thrill of a childhood adventure, or the triumph of a hard-earned success, our memories serve as both anchors and gateways, connecting us to the past while illuminating our path forward.

As we navigate the intricate landscape of memory, we gain a deeper understanding of its complexities and nuances, enriching our self-awareness and deepening our connection to the shared human experience. We come to appreciate the role that memory plays in shaping our emotions, guiding our decisions, and informing our perspectives. Through this exploration, we uncover the profound ways in which memory shapes our lives and our sense of who we are.

In essence, memory is the foundation upon which our identities are built. It is the repository of our experiences, the wellspring of our emotions, and the compass that guides us through life. By exploring its intricate layers and diverse forms, we come to appreciate the beauty and complexity of this mental tapestry and the vital role it plays in shaping our self-awareness and our understanding of the world.

CHAPTER 4

The Cognitive Benefits of Staying Active

In traversing the enigmatic corridors of human memory, we encounter an unanticipated ally in our quest for enduring recollection: the transformative power of physical movement. In its myriad forms, exercise serves not merely as a vessel for muscular or cardiovascular enhancement but as a sanctified arena where the mind can forge, fortify, and finesse its capacity to remember.

Staying physically active is more than just a good habit for your body; it's essential to fuel your brain as a protective shield against memory problems. Regular exercise—particularly aerobic activities like walking, running, or swimming—doesn't just work your muscles; it showers your brain with benefits that are too good to ignore.

Exercise acts as a natural booster for your brain in several significant ways. First, it increases blood flow to your brain, ensuring it receives the oxygen and nutrients needed to function at its best. This blood flow acts like a river of life for your brain cells, keeping them active and healthy.

Second, exercise enhances neuroplasticity, which is your brain's incredible ability to adapt, grow, and change throughout life. Imagine your brain as a city with many different roads. Neuroplasticity is like the construction crew that builds new roads and fixes old ones, helping you think more clearly and remember better.

Third, being active stimulates the growth of new brain cells, also known as neurons. Think of these as extra helpers in your brain that make it easier for you to store and retrieve memories, focus on tasks, and process information quickly.

But the benefits don't stop at your brain; they extend to your overall health. Regular physical activity helps control your blood sugar levels, reducing your risk of developing conditions like diabetes. This is important because high blood sugar problems can hurt your brain health over time.

In summary, an active lifestyle isn't just about staying fit and looking good; it's vital to keeping your brain sharp and effective. Exercise enriches your cognitive abilities, improving your thinking, remembering, and solving problems. It's like an investment in your future self, a gift that keeps on giving, enriching the quality of your life in countless ways. So, if you're looking for a compelling reason to get moving, consider this: your brain will thank you.

Cognitive Benefits of Regular Physical Exercise

Regular physical exercise does more than keep your body in shape; it's also a powerhouse for your brain. From boosting memory to enhancing focus, exercise offers a range of cognitive benefits that improve your thinking and overall mental well-being. Getting active can help you keep your mind sharp, and that's why it's imperative for brain health. So, let's get moving—your brain will thank you for it!

Enhanced Memory

Have you ever found yourself grappling with forgetfulness, straining to remember a name, or scrambling to recall an important detail? If so, you're not alone. Memory can be a fickle companion, often slipping away at the most inopportune moments. However, exercise is a powerful tool at your disposal that can help boost your memory and cognitive abilities.

Numerous research studies have demonstrated a consistent and compelling link between physical activity and improved memory. Regular exercise appears to enhance the brain's ability to encode, store, and retrieve information. In essence, when you work out your body, you also work out your brain, giving your memory a much-needed workout.

The benefits of exercise on memory are both immediate and long-lasting. In the short term, exercise increases blood flow to the brain, delivering a fresh supply of oxygen and nutrients that support cognitive function. Over time, regular physical activity stimulates the growth of new brain cells and strengthens existing neural connections, leading to improved memory and overall cognitive health.

Whether you're looking to remember names more effortlessly, recall to-do items, or simply feel more confident in your cognitive abilities, incorporating exercise into your routine can make a significant difference. The best part? You don't need to train for a marathon or become a bodybuilder to reap the benefits. Even moderate exercise, such as walking, cycling, or swimming, can yield positive results for your memory.

It's important to note that the relationship between exercise and memory is not merely anecdotal or based on a handful of studies. A growing body of scientific evidence supports this connection, with research showing that exercise promotes the growth of new neurons and improves overall brain health. For example, a study published in the journal "Neurobiology of Aging" found that older adults who engaged in regular physical activity had improved memory and cognitive function compared to those who did not exercise.

In addition to the direct benefits to memory, exercise also supports overall health and well-being, promoting better sleep, reducing stress, and improving mood. A healthier, more relaxed, and well-rested body creates a more favorable environment for memory formation and retrieval.

So, if you're looking to sharpen your memory and boost your cognitive abilities, consider making exercise a regular part of your routine. Even moderate physical activity can yield significant benefits, supporting memory and overall brain health. Remember, the brain, like any other muscle, benefits from a good workout.

Improved Attention

Exercise is not only a powerful tool for boosting memory but also for improving focus and attention. In today's fast-paced and distraction-filled world, the ability to concentrate and stay on task is more indispensable than ever. Fortunately, regular physical activity can help to strengthen your attention span and enhance your ability to focus on the task at hand.

Physical activities, particularly those that elevate your heart rate, have been shown to improve cognitive function, including focus and attention. As you engage in exercise, your brain is trained to become better at filtering out distractions and concentrating on the essential information. This improved ability to focus can translate to better performance in both work and everyday activities.

The benefits of exercise on focus and attention are particularly relevant in our current environment, where distractions are ubiquitous. From social media notifications to the constant influx of information, our attention is pulled in multiple directions. Exercise provides an effective way to counteract these challenges, helping to improve our cognitive control and sustain attention on important tasks.

So, the next time you find yourself struggling to concentrate or feeling your mind wander, consider incorporating physical activity into your day. A brisk walk, a quick run, or even a short workout can help clear your mind, sharpen your focus, and enhance your cognitive abilities. The key is to make exercise a regular habit, allowing your brain to reap the long-term benefits of improved focus, attention, and overall cognitive health.

In summary, the positive impact of exercise on cognitive function extends beyond memory enhancement to include focus and attention. Regular physical activity helps to condition the brain to filter distractions, concentrate on essential information, and sustain attention on important tasks. Incorporating exercise into your routine can help you combat the challenges of distraction and improve your cognitive abilities.

Faster Information Processing

Regular exercise not only strengthens memory and focus but also accelerates information processing. Just as upgrading the speed of a computer enhances its performance, regular physical activity can boost your brain's ability to rapidly absorb, process, and react to new information. This enhancement is not limited to cognitive tasks like problem-solving or decision-making but extends to everyday activities.

Research has consistently shown that individuals who engage in regular physical activity demonstrate faster information processing compared to those who are less active. This increased speed in information processing can be likened to upgrading the processing power of a computer. The upgraded system can handle more data and produce faster results, mirroring the improvement in cognitive function that occurs with regular exercise.

The impact of quicker information processing on everyday life is significant. Whether you're driving, working, or simply conversing with others, the ability to rapidly absorb, process, and react to new information provides a clear advantage. This heightened cognitive function allows you to make faster decisions, respond to situations more efficiently, and navigate life's challenges with greater ease.

Moreover, quicker information processing can enhance your performance in various activities, including sports, gaming, and creative pursuits. The enhanced speed of information processing enabled by regular exercise translates to improved reaction times, coordination, and overall performance.

The relationship between regular exercise and faster information processing is supported by scientific evidence, with research demonstrating that physical activity promotes brain health, enhances cognitive function, and protects against age-related cognitive decline. Incorporating exercise into your routine not only upgrades your brain's speed but also supports overall mental well-being, bolstering your ability to navigate the challenges of daily life.

In conclusion, the benefits of regular exercise extend beyond improved memory and focus to include accelerated information processing. This increased speed in cognitive function can provide a significant advantage in various aspects of life, from navigating everyday challenges to excelling in creative and physical pursuits. By incorporating exercise into your routine, you can effectively upgrade your brain's processing power, enhancing your ability to rapidly absorb, process, and react to new information.

Aerobic Exercise and Brain Health

Aerobic activities like walking, running, swimming, and cycling are particularly effective when boosting your brain's performance. One of the primary reasons is that these activities get your heart pumping, increasing blood flow throughout your body and brain.

This surge of blood delivers a cocktail of essential nutrients and oxygen that your brain cells need to function at their best. Think of it as a delivery service, where the better the circulation, the faster and more efficiently these vital supplies reach their destination, i.e., your brain cells.

But it's not just about supplying your brain with what it needs to function day-to-day. Aerobic exercise can enhance neuroplasticity, your brain's innate capacity to adapt, change, and grow over time. This adaptability is crucial for everything from learning new skills to recovering from injury.

The brain is continually rewiring itself, forming new connections between neurons. Aerobic exercise acts as a catalyst for this process, making it faster and more efficient. This improved neuroplasticity contributes significantly to your cognitive vitality, meaning you're better equipped to handle complex mental tasks, learn new information, and even fight off the cognitive decline of aging.

So, don't underestimate the power of aerobic activities when choosing a form of exercise with your cognitive well-being in mind. Whether going for a swim, enjoying a long bike ride, or just taking a brisk walk around the neighborhood, these exercises offer many brain-boosting benefits that contribute to a sharper, healthier you.

Reflections on The Cognitive Benefits of Staying Active

In a world increasingly driven by quick fixes and immediate gratification, exercise is a compelling testament to the enduring interplay between body and mind. To view exercise merely as a tool for physical enhancement is to ignore its profound cognitive advantages—a treasure trove of mental rewards that go hand in hand with noticeable physical gains.

When you commit to regular physical activity, you sculpt a stronger, more agile body and nurture a sharper, more resilient mind. With every heartbeat elevated through aerobic exercises like jogging, swimming, or cycling, a cascade of benefits showers your brain. From bolstering memory to improving your focus, exercise is the unsung hero in the realm of cognitive well-being.

Exercise serves as the custodian of this intricate system. It improves neuroplasticity, your brain's innate ability to adapt and evolve. This makes you more capable of learning new skills and equips you to face the evolving challenges that come with different life stages.

And let's not forget the role of exercise in mental health. Physical activity releases endorphins, the body's natural mood lifters. This has a cascade effect on your mental clarity and focus, offering you a natural shield against stress, anxiety, and even depression. The confidence gained from physical achievements often spills over into other areas of life, offering a renewed sense of purpose and self-efficacy.

Thus, the next time you tie your shoelaces for a run or put on your swimsuit for a swim, know that you're not just engaging in a physical routine. It's a ritual that honors your body and mind, benefiting and strengthening the other in a symbiotic relationship of well-being. Exercise is not just a good habit or a medical recommendation; it's a lifestyle, a philosophy, a statement you make to yourself: that you're worth the effort, now and for all the days to come.

CHAPTER 5

Nutrition for a Healthy Brain

Nutrition plays a pivotal role in enhancing memory and cognitive function. Essential nutrients act as the building blocks for healthy brain cells and the neural connections that support memory. Embracing a balanced diet rich in these nutrients can empower you to optimize your cognitive abilities and nurture a sharp and agile memory, promoting a positive and vibrant outlook on life.

A well-balanced diet is key for maintaining physical health and optimal brain function. As a highly metabolically active organ, the brain relies on a constant supply of nutrients to perform effectively. However, the realm of nutrition and diet is fraught with controversy and ongoing debates fueled by the complexity of these topics and evolving scientific research.

One of the enduring debates centers around low-carb diets versus low-fat diets, with conflicting studies regarding their effectiveness for weight loss and overall health. Plant-based diets have gained popularity, but concerns persist regarding the quality of animal products and their environmental impact. Intermittent fasting, often praised for its metabolic benefits, raises questions about the optimal fasting schedule and potential long-term effects.

Dietary supplements also spark controversy, with some advocating for filling nutrient gaps while others emphasize the superiority of whole foods. Debates surrounding sugar and artificial sweeteners continue, with ongoing discussions about their health implications. The role of saturated fat in heart health remains a subject of scrutiny. Personalized nutrition, although promising, faces challenges related to practicality and cost. Environmental considerations, such as the impact of meat production and food sustainability, add complexity to the ongoing dialogue.

In the ongoing discourse surrounding processed foods and their impact on human health, it is important to acknowledge that not all processed foods are inherently harmful. While some processed foods, such as those high in added sugars, sodium, and unhealthy fats, can contribute to various health issues, others may offer nutritional benefits or support convenient, time-saving meal options. For instance, certain canned fruits and vegetables, whole-grain cereals, and reduced-sodium soups are examples of processed foods that can fit into a balanced diet.

Navigating the complexities of food processing and nutrition requires a thoughtful and individualized approach. Staying informed about the latest research and consulting with healthcare professionals can help individuals make educated dietary choices that align with their unique health goals and needs. Balancing the potential benefits and drawbacks of processed foods with a focus on overall nutritional quality and personal well-being is essential for achieving long-term health and wellness.

A Dietary Guideline for Optimal Brain Health

In recent years, there has been an increased focus on understanding the impact of nutrition on brain health. Research suggests that certain foods and nutrients can influence cognitive function, mood, and the risk of neurological disorders. Incorporating these findings into dietary guidelines can help individuals optimize their brain health and reduce the risk of age-related cognitive decline and neurodegenerative diseases.

By following a dietary guideline tailored for optimal brain health, individuals can empower themselves to take control of their cognitive well-being and promote overall mental vitality.

Omega-3 Fatty Acids

Omega-3 fatty acids, specifically Eicosapentaenoic Acid (EPA) and Docosahexaenoic Acid (DHA) found in fatty fish like salmon, sardines, and mackerel, stand as vital components in the complex machinery of brain function. These essential fats are not merely optional supplements but imperative elements that actively sculpt the landscape of our neural architecture. Their role in reducing inflammation extends beyond alleviating bodily discomfort; they directly influence the brain's milieu by mitigating neuroinflammation, creating an environment conducive to efficient cognitive processes.

The story of Omega-3's positive impact doesn't end with controlling inflammation. These fats are linchpins in supporting neuronal communication, the essential exchange of information between nerve cells at the heart of all cognitive functions. By aiding in forming cellular membranes and acting as modulators in neurotransmitter systems, Omega-3 fatty acids ensure that messages between neurons are transferred swiftly and accurately.

36

Furthermore, EPA and DHA also contribute to neurogenesis—the formation of new neurons—especially in the hippocampus, a region of the brain intricately linked with memory and spatial navigation. Regular consumption of these fatty acids thus becomes an act of proactive brain health maintenance, enhancing both memory and a broad array of cognitive abilities. In integrating Omega-3-rich foods into one's diet or via supplementation under medical guidance, individuals may invest in their present well-being and secure the resilience and vitality of their minds for the future.

Antioxidant-Rich Foods

Antioxidants, frequently celebrated for their role in skincare and general well-being, have a transformative impact on cognitive health that is both deep and enduring. These potent compounds are primarily found in a colorful array of fruits and vegetables, including but not limited to blueberries, strawberries, and blackberries. These berries are not just culinary delights; they're veritable powerhouses of cognitive enhancement, brimming with antioxidants like anthocyanins and flavonoids.

One of the most critical battles these antioxidants wage is against oxidative stress, a biochemical imbalance that accelerates cellular aging and decay. Oxidative stress can erode neurons' structural integrity and functionality within the brain, contributing to cognitive decline and memory loss over time. By neutralizing free radicals, which are oxidative stress agents, antioxidants help maintain brain cells' structural integrity, thereby prolonging their efficacy.

Another front where antioxidants assert their influence is in the mitigation of inflammation. Chronic inflammation can act as a silent but relentless aggressor, impairing cognitive functions by creating a hostile neural environment. Antioxidants serve as biochemical peacekeepers, calming this inflammatory turmoil and restoring balance and tranquility to the neural landscape.

Various scientific studies have linked compounds in these antioxidant-rich foods, particularly anthocyanins and flavonoids, to enhanced memory and cognitive function. These compounds protect neural structures and facilitate better communication between neurons. This results in more efficient brain function, improving memory, attention, and problem-solving skills.

So, incorporating antioxidant-rich foods into your diet is more than a lifestyle choice; it's a strategic maneuver to defend, sustain, and elevate your cognitive capabilities. Consuming these fruits and vegetables is an investment in your physical health and a long-term commitment to preserving and enhancing your mental acuity.

Whole Grains

Whole grains, often lauded for their benefits to digestive health and heart well-being, offer a nuanced contribution to cognitive functioning that can be subtle and profound. Staple foods like oatmeal, brown rice, and quinoa go beyond mere components of a balanced diet; they serve as a refined energy delivery system for the brain. Unlike processed grains, which may lead to rapid spikes and subsequent crashes in blood sugar levels, whole grains facilitate a more stable and steady release of glucose into the bloodstream.

This consistent glucose flow functions like a well-tuned energy supply for the brain, ensuring it operates at peak efficiency for extended periods. The brain is an energy-intensive organ, requiring a constant fuel source to manage its myriad tasks, from basic survival functions to complex cognitive processes like decision-making and problem-solving. A steady glucose supply thus becomes tantamount to having a dependable and long-lasting energy reservoir that keeps the brain vigilant and focused.

This sustained energy promotes prolonged concentration and helps maintain a state of mental alertness throughout the day. The ramifications are broad-reaching, from enhanced productivity in task-oriented activities to improved performance in intellectual or creative endeavors. Moreover, a steady fuel source could mitigate the typical afternoon slump many people experience, providing a baseline energy level that prevents cognitive fatigue.

In the broader context, incorporating whole grains into one's dietary habits is akin to making a long-term investment in mental wellness. The benefits manifest in immediate tasks and accumulate over time, potentially staving off cognitive decline and enhancing overall brain function.

Lean Proteins

Lean proteins, often associated with muscle building and metabolic support, are underappreciated yet pivotal in shaping and sustaining cognitive health. Sources such as chicken, fish, and tofu are not merely components of a nutritious meal; they are foundational blocks that support the biochemical intricacies of the brain. Proteins break down into amino acids, the raw material for synthesizing neurotransmitters like serotonin, dopamine, and norepinephrine. These neurotransmitters act as chemical messengers facilitating communication across neural networks, ensuring the brain functions smoothly and efficiently. Serotonin is often called the "feel-good" neurotransmitter, integral to regulating mood, sleep, and appetite. Dopamine, on the other hand, is commonly associated with the pleasure and reward system but also plays a significant role in attention and focus. Norepinephrine works with dopamine and affects alertness, arousal, and reaction speed. These neurotransmitters create a finely tuned symphony that influences how we feel, think, learn, and remember.

Incorporating lean proteins into one's diet ensures a consistent supply of these essential amino acids, guaranteeing that neurotransmitter levels remain balanced. This biochemical equilibrium translates into more stable mood patterns, heightened mental clarity, and overall well-being. A steady influx of these proteins helps ward off the emotional highs and lows accompanying an imbalanced diet, leading to a more focused and stable cognitive state.

Therefore, lean proteins are a dietary choice and a strategic element in the quest for cognitive excellence and emotional stability. Including them in your diet becomes an act of self-care that goes beyond physical wellness, enveloping the mind in a protective cloak of biochemical resilience. As part of a balanced diet, lean proteins offer a pathway to enhanced mental function, emotional balance, and long-term cognitive vitality.

Healthy Fats

Healthy fats, often branded as "good fats," are paramount in maintaining and elevating cognitive health. Specifically, monounsaturated fats found in nourishing foods like avocados and olive oil are far more than just heart-healthy choices; they are integral to the brain's structural and functional well-being. These fats contribute to forming and maintaining brain cell membranes, serving as both guardians and facilitators for these essential neural structures.

Brain cell membranes are not passive barriers but dynamic interfaces that regulate the flow of nutrients, ions, and information in and out of the cell. The integrity of these membranes is Important for their role as gatekeepers of cellular activity, ensuring that each neuron can function at its peak potential. A compromised membrane could lead to inefficient communication between brain cells, adversely affecting cognitive functions like memory and learning.

Monounsaturated fats bolster this cellular architecture, enhancing the fluidity and flexibility of these membranes. In doing so, they facilitate more efficient communication between neurons. Efficient neural communication is the linchpin of all cognitive activities, from the encoding and retrieval of memories to complex problem-solving and emotional regulation.

By incorporating these healthy fats into your daily nutritional regimen, you're not merely adhering to a balanced diet but also actively promoting optimal brain function. This influence extends from immediate cognitive performance enhancements to potentially delaying age-related cognitive decline. In essence, including monounsaturated fats in your diet is not just a dietary preference but a conscious, strategic decision to nurture and sustain mental acuity and cognitive resilience throughout life.

B Vitamins

B vitamins constitute a complex family, each serving a unique yet synergistic role in brain health and memory function. The most prominent among these for cognitive wellness are B1 (Thiamine), B3 (Niacin), B6 (Pyridoxine), B9 (Folic Acid or Folate), and B12 (Cobalamin).

Thiamine (B1) is involved in glucose metabolism, the brain's primary energy source. A thiamine deficiency can lead to issues with memory and cognitive function. Niacin (B3) is essential for DNA repair and the production of stress-related hormones, playing a part in maintaining the health of brain cells. Pyridoxine (B6) is a coenzyme in the metabolism of amino acids, the building blocks of proteins and neurotransmitters, thus having a direct impact on memory and other cognitive processes.

Then comes Folic Acid or Folate (B9), essential in synthesizing neurotransmitters and DNA and RNA synthesis, affecting cell growth and gene expression. A folate deficiency is linked to elevated levels of homocysteine, which has been correlated with cognitive decline and a variety of neurodegenerative diseases. Finally, Cobalamin (B12) is vital for maintaining the health of the nervous system and is involved in creating red blood cells, which carry oxygen to the brain. Like B9, B12 also plays a role in regulating homocysteine levels.

Each of these B vitamins has its source of food. Thiamine is commonly found in whole grains, legumes, meats, and fish. Niacin is abundant in animal products like meat, fish, legumes, and nuts. Pyridoxine is present in various foods, including meat, dairy, and certain vegetables like carrots and spinach. Folate can be sourced from leafy greens, legumes, and fortified cereals. Cobalamin is mainly found in animal products, making it essential for vegetarians and vegans to seek alternative sources or supplements.

Incorporating a diverse range of these B vitamins into your diet becomes a multifaceted strategy for optimizing memory function. Each vitamin contributes its unique strengths, building a composite picture of cognitive wellness that is more than the sum of its parts. The B vitamin complex provides a robust shield against memory decline, offering immediate and long-term cognitive benefits.

Hydration

Dehydration, often subtly dismissed as a minor concern, carries significant implications for cognitive function, particularly in attention and memory. When the body lacks sufficient hydration, it doesn't merely affect physical stamina or skin health; it also creates an environment where mental faculties are compromised.

Specifically, dehydration can manifest as a noticeable hindrance in one's ability to concentrate, making tasks that require sustained focus considerably more challenging. Even more critically, dehydration can impair memory retrieval, causing a struggle to recall basic information.

This is because water plays an indispensable role in the biochemical processes that enable our neurons to communicate effectively with each other. These processes become less efficient without adequate hydration, affecting our cognitive abilities. The amount of water a person should drink can vary based on various factors such as age, sex, weight, activity level, and even the climate in which they live. However, a general guideline often cited is to drink eight 8-ounce glasses of water daily, commonly known as the "8x8 rule," which amounts to about half a gallon or approximately two liters.

However, some health experts recommend a more individualized approach, suggesting you drink at least half an ounce to an ounce of water for each pound you weigh. For example, weighing 150 pounds, you might aim for 75 to 150 ounces of water daily. Athletes or those who live in hot climates may need even more.

It's also important to consider other sources of water intake, including food (fruits and vegetables can have high water content) and other beverages. However, it's advisable to limit beverages high in sugar or caffeine, as they can lead to dehydration.

Lastly, it's essential to listen to your body. Thirst is an obvious sign to drink more, but other indicators like the color of your urine can also be a helpful gauge. Light yellow or clear urine usually indicates good hydration. In contrast, a darker yellow or amber color might mean you need more water.

Always consult with a healthcare provider for the most accurate health advice.

Limit Processed Foods

Processed foods, often considered convenient and palatable, carry a hidden cost, particularly regarding cognitive health. These foods are typically laden with unhealthy fats, refined sugars, and a cocktail of additives, ranging from preservatives to flavor enhancers. While these ingredients may extend shelf life or enhance taste, they promote inflammation and oxidative stress within the brain. Inflammation and oxidative stress are not merely abstract biochemical events; they are powerful agents that can negatively impact brain cells, affecting the neural pathways vital for memory, decision-making, and other cognitive functions.

The connection between inflammation and cognitive function is increasingly becoming a focal point in neuroscience research. Inflammation disrupts the delicate balance of neurotransmitters and can cause a chain reaction of damaging effects, from disrupting the brain's protective barrier to killing off neurons. Similarly, oxidative stress damages the cellular structure, contributing to aging and the risk of degenerative diseases like Alzheimer's and Parkinson's.

Against this backdrop, reducing the consumption of processed foods isn't just a dietary adjustment; it's a strategic move aimed at mitigating risk factors linked to cognitive decline. A shift towards whole, unprocessed foods represents more than a change in grocery shopping habits. It is a commitment to nourish the brain with the essential nutrients it needs to perform optimally.

Whole, unprocessed foods are often rich in antioxidants, healthy fats, fiber, and an array of vitamins and minerals, all of which contribute to a well-balanced biochemical environment for the brain. Foods like fruits, vegetables, lean proteins, and whole grains offer diverse nutrients that counteract the damaging effects of inflammation and oxidative stress, creating a protective buffer for cognitive health.

Opting for whole, unprocessed foods over their processed counterparts is akin to choosing a path of cognitive resilience. This decision supports immediate brain function and offers a long-term investment in preserving mental acuity and overall well-being. It's a choice that transcends momentary pleasure, emphasizing a lifetime of cognitive vitality and health.

Drink Alcohol in Moderation

Moderate alcohol consumption, according to some studies, may have specific cognitive benefits. However, excessive alcohol intake is detrimental to memory and cognitive function. It's essential to adhere to recommended limits, which typically means up to one drink per day for women and up to two drinks per day for men. This level of alcohol intake is generally considered safe. It offers certain cardiovascular benefits while minimizing the potential harm to cognitive health.

The subject of alcohol's role in cognitive health is a multi-faceted one, teetering between potential benefits and significant risks. Some scientific studies have suggested that moderate alcohol consumption may have particular cognitive advantages, such as a reduced risk for dementia, and certain cardiovascular benefits, such as improved blood flow. Cardiovascular improvements, in turn, could indirectly positively affect brain health by ensuring a steady supply of oxygen and nutrients to this critical organ. Yet, it's key to emphasize that these benefits are associated with moderate consumption—usually as up to one drink per day for women and up to two drinks per day for men.

However, the dark side of alcohol consumption should not be overlooked. Excessive drinking can severely impair memory and cognitive function in the short- and long-term. It can lead to cognitive deficits, affecting attention, decision-making, and problem-solving processes. Over time, heavy alcohol consumption can lead to neurodegeneration, contributing to long-term issues like dementia and other neurocognitive disorders. Alcohol can also interact negatively with medications and exacerbate existing health conditions, making it a risky choice for some individuals regardless of the amount consumed.

This dual nature of alcohol makes adhering to recommended guidelines vital. Staying within these recommended limits offers a level of safety, minimizing alcohol's negative cognitive impact while potentially reaping some of its cardiovascular benefits. Yet it's essential to consult with healthcare providers to consider your unique health profile, including any medications you are taking or other medical conditions you may have.

While moderate alcohol consumption may offer some cognitive and cardiovascular benefits, the operative word is "moderate." Crossing that boundary into excessive consumption can lead to significant cognitive impairments and negate any potential benefits. Therefore, it's crucial to approach alcohol consumption cautiously, aware of its potential benefits and substantial risks.

The Role of Glucose and Lactate

The relationship between what we eat and how our brain functions is an area of growing interest and research. Specifically, glucose and lactate—two types of sugar—play critical roles in memory formation and recall. As we dive into the science behind it, you'll better understand why glucose and lactate are more than just fuel for the body; they're essential players in maintaining a sharp and effective memory.

Glucose as Brain Fuel

When it comes to powering the complex machinery of our brains, glucose is a key player. It's a specific type of sugar that our bodies obtain from carbohydrates. While we might often hear about the potential dangers of consuming too much sugar, it's essential to remember that in moderate amounts, glucose is the primary fuel for our brains, especially at rest. Our brains are incredibly energy-hungry, consuming about 20% of our body's total energy, and glucose helps to meet this demand. This energy sustains the myriad of cellular activities in our brain at any given moment, supporting everything from essential functions like breathing and heart rate to more complex tasks like decision-making and memory retention.

Lactate Production during Exercise

When you engage in physical exercise, especially aerobic types like running or swimming, your body begins consuming glucose reserves for energy. As this happens, your brain produces lactate, a byproduct or metabolite of this energy conversion process. Contrary to some older theories that painted lactate as a waste product, modern research shows that lactate serves beneficial roles. It is imperative for driving metabolism and contributes to various health benefits. Lactate isn't just a footnote in the energy conversion process; it's a valuable contributor to your well-being.

Enhanced Cerebral Blood Flow (CBF)

One of the most exciting aspects of lactate production during exercise is its impact on cerebral blood flow, commonly known by its abbreviation, CBF. As lactate levels rise during physical activity, they trigger an increase in the flow of blood to your brain. This is a game-changer for brain efficiency. Enhanced blood flow ensures that your brain is continually supplied with the nutrients and oxygen required for optimal function. It's like upgrading the supply chain for a factory, allowing it to produce goods more efficiently and effectively. In the context of your brain, this translates to improved cognitive performance, making tasks that require focus, quick thinking, and memory recall easier to manage.

Glucose and lactate support brain function and improve cognitive abilities like memory. While glucose is the primary energy source at rest, lactate takes the stage during exercise, each contributing to the complex and fascinating interplay of nutrients fueling our minds.

Reflections on Nutrition for a Healthy Brain

The dietary choices we make not only impact our individual cognitive function and physical health but also contribute to the broader socio-cultural and environmental context. As we navigate ongoing debates in nutrition science, it is important to recognize that this field is a constantly evolving landscape. Despite the differing opinions, there are certain universal guidelines that remain relevant and essential for promoting overall well-being.

One such guideline is the importance of Omega-3 fatty acids in supporting cognitive function. These essential fats, found in fatty fish, walnuts, and flax seeds, play a critical role in brain development and function. Additionally, staying hydrated is a fundamental aspect of maintaining optimal physical and cognitive performance. Dehydration can negatively impact mood, energy levels, and cognitive function, underscoring the importance of drinking adequate water throughout the day.

A holistic perspective on diet and cognitive function recognizes that individual nutrients and dietary choices are interconnected with other lifestyle factors. For instance, physical activity and dietary sugars like glucose and lactate interact to influence memory formation and cerebral blood flow. These interactions highlight the interdependence of dietary choices, physical activity, and cognitive health, emphasizing the importance of a comprehensive approach to well-being.

As the conversation around diet evolves, sustainability considerations and environmental impact have become increasingly important. The foods we choose have implications for both our individual health and the health of the planet. Adopting a sustainable diet that is nutritionally balanced, diverse, and environmentally conscious is essential for promoting both personal and planetary well-being.

In this complex landscape, the key takeaway remains that making informed, balanced nutritional choices is essential for both physical and mental health. By considering the interconnectedness of diet, lifestyle, and environmental factors, we can promote a holistic approach to well-being that supports individual cognitive function and contributes to a more sustainable future.

CHAPTER 6

Sleep's Impact on Memory

Sleep is a cornerstone for cognitive function, particularly regarding memory retention and consolidation. During the various stages of sleep, our brains work tirelessly to sift through the plethora of information we've encountered throughout the day. This intricate process allows us to recall information more effectively, making sleep a critical factor in learning, problem-solving, and emotional well-being. Missing adequate sleep can disrupt these key processes, diminishing memory and cognitive performance.

A good night's sleep is a cognitive powerhouse, impacting memory, creativity, and emotional stability. During sleep, the brain consolidates memories, transforming short-term into long-term, enhancing learning capacity. Rapid Eye Movement (REM) sleep fosters creativity and problem-solving, generating innovative ideas. Sleep also regulates emotions; restful sleep stabilizes mood, while deprivation can lead to irritability and anxiety. Sleep detoxifies the brain as the glymphatic system flushes out toxins, which is essential for cognitive function. It enhances attention and focus, improving productivity. Adequate sleep is indispensable for overall mental health. Chronic sleep deprivation increases the risk of cognitive decline, including Alzheimer's. Prioritizing sleep and maintaining good sleep hygiene are both vital for preserving cognitive abilities as we age.

What Does a Good Night's Sleep Do?

A good night's sleep is often heralded as the cornerstone of a healthy lifestyle. Yet, many people still underestimate its true importance. While it's common knowledge that sleep helps us feel refreshed, its more profound impact on our physical and mental well-being is less widely discussed.

From enhancing cognitive function to fortifying the immune system, the benefits of quality sleep are manifold. So, what exactly does a good night's sleep do for us? Let's unravel the science behind sleep and its indispensable role in our lives.

Cognitive Processes

Sleep is like a backstage crew working diligently to make sense of the day's events. During this downtime, our brains process and organize the information we've encountered, creating the foundation for memory formation and retaining new knowledge. Imagine it as a librarian carefully cataloging and shelving books. When we skimp on sleep, this cognitive work is compromised, leading to learning, memory recall, and problem-solving difficulties. The mental clutter accumulates, making finding the information we need challenging.

Attention and Focus

Think of sleep as an orchestra conductor. When we enjoy a good night's rest, our attention and focus are finely tuned, allowing us to stay alert and responsive. But when sleep is disrupted or inadequate, it's as if the orchestra is out of tune, resulting in slower reaction times, difficulty concentrating on tasks at work or school, and a general feeling of mental fogginess.

Mood Regulation

Sleep and emotions are intricately connected, like a seesaw in a playground. When we don't get enough sleep, it's as if one side of the seesaw is weighed down, leading to mood disturbances. Irritability, mood swings, and heightened susceptibility to stress and anxiety become more prevalent. The seesaw becomes imbalanced, and we struggle to maintain emotional equilibrium. Moreover, insufficient sleep can exacerbate symptoms of depression, making it even more important to prioritize restful slumber for our overall emotional well-being.

The Glymphatic System and Sleep

One fascinating discovery in sleep and brain health is the glymphatic system, a relatively recent addition to our understanding of brain function. This system operates as a macroscopic waste clearance mechanism within the brain, akin to a diligent janitorial crew working overnight to clean up the day's mess. It accomplishes this essential task through a network of perivascular channels formed by specialized brain cells known as astroglial cells. These cells are the channels through which waste products, including harmful proteins and metabolites, are efficiently removed from the central nervous system. During these restful hours, the brain can effectively clear the clutter and prepare for another day of learning, problem-solving, and memory consolidation.

Creating Healthy Sleep Habits

Healthy sleep habits, often called sleep hygiene, are essential for ensuring restorative and restful sleep. Establishing and maintaining these habits can significantly improve the quality of your sleep and overall well-being. Here are some healthy sleep habits to consider:

Consistent Sleep Schedule

Maintaining a consistent sleep schedule is like setting the body's internal clock to the correct time zone. Just as a synchronized watch keeps accurate time, going to bed and waking up simultaneously each day helps regulate your body's circadian rhythm, making it easier to fall asleep and wake up feeling refreshed. This consistency strengthens your body's internal cues for when it's time to rest, promoting a healthier sleep pattern.

Create a Comfortable Sleep Environment

Your bedroom should be your sleep sanctuary, where relaxation and tranquility rule. Think of it as creating the perfect stage for a good night's sleep. Invest in a comfortable mattress and pillows that provide the necessary support for your body. Ensure that your room is dark, quiet, and comfortably cool, typically between 60 and 67 degrees Fahrenheit (15 to 19 degrees Celsius), replicating the ideal sleeping conditions in nature.

Limit Exposure to Screens

The digital age has brought an abundance of screens, from smartphones to tablets and televisions. While these devices offer countless conveniences, their blue light emissions can disrupt the body's production of melatonin, the hormone responsible for regulating sleep.

Avoiding electronic devices at least an hour before bedtime allows your melatonin levels to rise naturally, helping you fall asleep more easily and enjoy a deeper, more restorative slumber.

Mind Your Diet

Much like fueling a car, the type and timing of your meals can affect your sleep. Large meals, caffeine, and alcohol close to bedtime can disrupt sleep. Instead, opt for a light, nutritious snack if you're hungry before bed. Consider foods rich in tryptophan, like a banana or a small serving of turkey, which can promote the production of sleep-inducing serotonin.

Regular Exercise

Physical activity is like a natural sleep aid, helping you drift into dreamland more easily—however, the timing of exercise matters. While regular physical activity promotes better sleep, avoid intense workouts close to bedtime, as they can rev up your metabolism and make it harder to fall asleep. Exercise earlier in the day to reap its sleep-enhancing benefits.

Relaxation Techniques

Relaxation is akin to soothing the mind before sleep. As you wind down after a busy day, take time to unwind your thoughts before bedtime. Techniques like deep breathing, meditation, and progressive muscle relaxation can calm the mind, reduce anxiety, and prepare you for a restful night's sleep.

Limit Naps

Napping can be a delightful afternoon escape, like a short vacation for your mind. However, napping for extended periods or too late in the day can disrupt your body's sleep-wake cycle. To avoid interfering with nighttime sleep, keep naps short (around 20-30 minutes) and schedule them earlier, ideally in the late morning or early afternoon.

Manage Stress

In the theater of the mind, stress can be a relentless performer, stealing the spotlight with its dazzling display of anxiety and concern. Its adeptness at keeping you awake at night is akin to a thunderstorm, with bolts of worry and apprehension illuminating the darkness. To navigate this turbulence and arrive at the tranquil shores of restful sleep, it's essential to cultivate effective stress management techniques.

Mindfulness serves as a beacon in the tempestuous sea of stress. By focusing on the present moment and acknowledging your thoughts and feelings without judgment, you can begin to cultivate a sense of calm and equilibrium. Journaling, too, can be a powerful ally in the fight against stress. By pouring your concerns onto paper, you're externalizing your worries, making them more manageable and less overwhelming.

Limit Liquid Intake Before Bed

Sipping a glass of water can be refreshing during the day, but too much liquid before bedtime can lead to midnight bathroom trips. To minimize disruptions to your sleep, reduce your liquid intake in the hours leading up to bedtime.

Expose Yourself to Natural Light

The sun is nature's timekeeper, guiding our internal clocks. Exposure to natural light during the day helps regulate your circadian rhythm, the body's natural sleep-wake cycle. Spend time outdoors during daylight hours and consider opening curtains or blinds to let natural light into your home, reinforcing your body's understanding of when it's time to be awake and when it's time to rest.

Establish a Bedtime Routine

A bedtime routine is like a soothing lullaby for your mind and body. Create a calming activity sequence that signals your brain that it's time to wind down and prepare for sleep. This could involve reading a book, taking a warm bath, or practicing relaxation exercises. By consistently following this routine, you condition your body to expect sleep and promote better sleep quality.

Limit Clock Watching

As the minutes tick away, checking the clock can morph into a source of anxiety about being unable to sleep. Instead of staring at the clock, try to relax. If sleep remains elusive, it's better to get out of bed and engage in a quiet, non-stimulating activity until you feel sleepy. This helps break the cycle of frustration and anxiety associated with trying to force sleep.

Seek Professional Help

While incorporating exercise, maintaining a sleep schedule, creating a restful environment, and practicing relaxation techniques can improve your sleep quality, it's essential to recognize when additional help is necessary. If you find that you're consistently struggling with sleep despite your best efforts, it's critical to seek the guidance of a healthcare professional or a sleep specialist.

Sleep disorders such as insomnia, sleep apnea, and restless legs syndrome can significantly impact sleep quality and duration. These conditions often require specialized treatments, including cognitive-behavioral therapy for insomnia, continuous positive airway pressure therapy for sleep apnea, or medication for restless legs syndrome. A healthcare professional or sleep specialist can diagnose any underlying sleep disorders and recommend an appropriate treatment plan tailored to your unique needs.

Seeking expert guidance not only helps you address potential sleep disorders but also supports your overall health and well-being. Persistent sleep issues can contribute to a variety of physical and mental health problems, including an increased risk of cardiovascular disease, diabetes, and mental health disorders like depression and anxiety. By seeking professional help, you can address these potential issues early and take proactive steps to support your health.

Moreover, working with a healthcare professional or sleep specialist allows you to develop a comprehensive sleep plan that incorporates lifestyle modifications, stress management techniques, and medical interventions, if necessary. This holistic approach ensures that you receive the tailored support you need to achieve restorative sleep and optimize your overall health.

Reflections on Sleep's Impact on Memory

Sleep, that sweet symphony of slumber, is more than just a restorative escape from the hustle and bustle of daily life. It is a fundamental pillar of our overall well-being, a conductor orchestrating the intricate ballet of our cognitive and emotional experiences. One of the lesser-known yet utterly essential roles that sleep plays is its involvement in the delicate process of memory consolidation.

As we drift off into the realm of dreams, our brains embark on a journey of organization and assimilation, sifting through the day's events, learnings, and experiences. It is during this nocturnal adventure that memories are meticulously curated, filed away into the labyrinthine corridors of our mind, awaiting retrieval at a moment's notice. This process, known as memory consolidation, is an indispensable cog in the wheel of cognitive function, allowing us to remember, learn, and adapt to the ever-changing canvas of life.

The magic of memory consolidation unfolds during various stages of sleep, with rapid eye movement (REM) and slow-wave sleep taking center stage. During REM sleep, our brains consolidate procedural and spatial memories, the building blocks of complex physical and navigational skills. Slow-wave sleep, on the other hand, works its magic on declarative memories, the repository of facts, events, and personal experiences. In a harmonious partnership, these stages of sleep collaborate to forge a robust and reliable memory network, enabling us to navigate the intricacies of life with ease and efficiency.

Yet, the importance of sleep for memory consolidation goes beyond the nightly routine. It serves as a stark reminder of the detrimental consequences of sleep deprivation. When we skimp on sleep, we're not just forfeiting a sense of refreshment; we're jeopardizing our cognitive abilities. A lack of sufficient sleep leaves us feeling sluggish and irritable, with our capacity to form and retrieve memories compromised. Over time, chronic sleep deprivation can cast a shadow over our long-term memory, contributing to cognitive decline and increased susceptibility to memory-related disorders.

In essence, the humble act of sleeping is a vital pillar supporting the edifice of our cognitive and emotional lives. It is the quiet hero, orchestrating the delicate balance between memory formation and retrieval, providing the bedrock for our mental agility and adaptability. So, the next time we slip into the embrace of sleep, let us remember that we are embarking on a journey of memory consolidation, strengthening the sinews of our mind and paving the way for a vibrant, fulfilling life.

CHAPTER 7

The Importance of Continuous Learning

One often overlooked strategy to combat cognitive decline is the practice of continuous learning. Mental stimulation can keep the mind sharp in our formative and peak productive years, but it is less discussed later in life. Can taking up a new hobby, learning a new language, or even engaging in regular intellectual discussions fortify the brain against the ravages of time? It's never too late to teach an old brain new tricks.

The importance of continuous learning in memory loss cannot be overstated. Learning new skills, acquiring knowledge, and engaging in intellectually stimulating activities are like exercises for the brain. They challenge the mind, promote neural connections, and enhance cognitive reserve. Our brains naturally change as we age, and memory decline concerns many. However, research suggests that individuals actively seeking opportunities to learn and challenge their cognitive abilities can significantly delay the onset of memory problems. This cognitive engagement strengthens memory and fosters neuroplasticity, allowing the brain to adapt and reorganize itself. It's a proactive approach to preserving memory and cognitive function, demonstrating that pursuing knowledge is a powerful tool in the fight against memory loss. Engaging in mentally stimulating activities is a powerful way to enhance brain health and cognitive abilities. Let's explore this concept further:

Benefits of Mentally Stimulating Activities

Engaging in mentally stimulating activities is enjoyable and imperative for brain health and cognitive abilities. Let's delve deeper into why these activities are so beneficial:

Cognitive Challenge

You work out your brain when you tackle puzzles, read, learn new skills, or play musical instruments. These activities require problem-solving, critical thinking, and creativity, challenging

54

different aspects of your cognitive function. For example, puzzles like crosswords or Sudoku stimulate logical reasoning, while playing a musical instrument can tap into your creativity and coordination.

Neurological Benefits

Engaging in these activities triggers complex processes in your brain. As you read a book or solve a puzzle, your brain's neurons fire and connect in intricate patterns. These connections strengthen neural pathways, allowing information to flow more efficiently. This not only improves memory but also enhances overall cognitive function.

Cognitive Reserve Building

Think of cognitive reserve as your brain's resilience. Just as physical exercise strengthens your muscles, mentally stimulating activities build cognitive reserve. This reserve protects against cognitive decline and neurological diseases such as Alzheimer's. So, the more you challenge your brain throughout your life, the better equipped it is to withstand age-related changes.

Neuroplasticity in Action

Neuroplasticity, often called the brain's ability to "rewire" itself, is remarkable. It means your brain can adapt and reorganize its structure in response to learning and experiences. Engaging in intellectually stimulating activities is like giving your brain tools to remodel itself. Your brain reshapes its neural networks as you learn new skills or take on cognitive challenges, fostering growth and adaptability.

Incorporating these activities into your daily routine keeps your mind sharp and enriches your life. Whether learning a new language, practicing a musical instrument, or tackling a challenging puzzle, your brain benefits from mental gymnastics, ensuring it stays agile and resilient throughout your lifetime.

Technology and Cognitive Benefits

Indeed, technology, often regarded as a double-edged sword, holds remarkable cognitive advantages, especially for older adults. It's intriguing to delve into how technology can serve as a valuable and transformative tool for enhancing cognitive abilities in this demographic. As we embark on this exploration, we'll uncover how technology can contribute to mental sharpness, problem-solving skills, and overall cognitive well-being among older individuals.

Brain Stimulation

Engaging with technology, from computers to smartphones, provides more than just practical benefits or entertainment; it also offers a valuable opportunity for mental exercise. Learning to navigate different digital platforms and apps and playing intellectually stimulating digital games can uniquely challenge our cognitive skills. These activities require a range of mental faculties, including memory, problem-solving, and logical thinking. As such, technology can act as a tool for keeping our minds sharp and improving our problem-solving abilities. However, it's important to use technology mindfully, balancing its cognitive benefits with the potential downsides of excessive or passive use.

Access to Information

Technology has fundamentally changed how we access information, offering a precious resource for older adults. The Internet breaks down traditional barriers to education and personal development, such as geographical distance or physical limitations, by providing a wealth of educational resources that can be accessed from home. This ease of access supports continuous learning, which is critical for cognitive health. Older adults can exercise necessary cognitive skills like problem-solving, indispensable thinking, and analytical reasoning by exploring new topics or hobbies online. While balancing screen time with other activities is critical, technology undeniably offers older adults a unique opportunity to enrich their intellectual lives and bolster their cognitive well-being.

Social Connectivity

Staying socially connected is important for mental well-being, especially as people age. Through social media platforms, video calls, and messaging apps, technology allows older adults to maintain and expand their social networks. Regular communication with friends and family can positively impact mood and cognitive function.

Cognitive Training Apps

The marketplace for cognitive training applications is rapidly expanding, reflecting a societal awareness of the importance of mental fitness. These apps target a range of cognitive abilities, including memory, attention, and problem-solving skills, and they are often built on principles derived from neuroscience and psychology. The interactive nature of these applications makes them particularly appealing; they frequently feature a variety of games and exercises specifically designed to challenge and stimulate different aspects of cognition.

While the scientific consensus on the long-term effectiveness of these apps is still a matter of ongoing research, preliminary studies have shown promising results for specific populations, such as older adults or individuals recovering from brain injuries. Even if the jury is still out on their efficacy, these apps offer an engaging, enjoyable way to keep the mind active, much like physical exercise for the brain.

Users also appreciate the flexibility and accessibility of these apps. They can be used anywhere and anytime, providing an easy way to incorporate cognitive training into daily routines. Many apps even offer progress-tracking features, allowing users to monitor their advancement and adjust their training accordingly. This personalized approach to cognitive stimulation can complement other forms of mental and physical activity, offering a multi-faceted approach to cognitive health.

Assistive Technology

Assistive technologies like reminder apps, digital calendars, and voice-activated devices are increasingly beneficial for people facing cognitive challenges or seeking to improve their organizational skills. Reminder apps help automate essential tasks, sending alerts for medications, appointments, or daily chores, thus reducing the mental burden of remembering everything. Digital calendars go a step further by providing an integrated system for tracking personal and shared events, easily syncing with other devices to keep everyone on the same page. Voice-activated devices offer hands-free utility, allowing users to perform various tasks through simple voice commands. These practical and user-friendly tools make life more manageable and provide peace of mind, regardless of age or tech-savvy.

Digital Hobbies

Technology integration into daily life has opened up many new opportunities for creative expression, and older adults are increasingly tapping into this resource. Many are discovering hobbies intrinsically linked to technology, such as digital photography, digital art creation, or even writing and publishing online.

Digital photography, for instance, goes beyond just snapping pictures with a smartphone or digital camera. Older adults can learn about the nuances of lighting, composition, and editing, transforming a simple photograph into a piece of art. This hobby enhances technical skills and sharpens observational abilities and aesthetic judgment.

Similarly, digital art platforms offer an accessible avenue for older adults to explore their artistic tendencies. With various programs and apps that simulate different art mediums—like watercolors, oils, or charcoal—individuals can create intricate artworks without the need for physical materials. The digital medium allows easy correction and experimentation, making the creative process less intimidating and inviting.

Writing, too, has been transformed by technology. With word processing software, older adults interested in penning their thoughts, stories, or expertise can easily do so. They can even publish their works through blogs or eBooks. Writing can serve as a significant cognitive exercise involving the formation of coherent sentences and paragraphs and the organization of thoughts and ideas into a structured narrative.

These creative outlets offer more than just a fun pastime; they provide tangible mental benefits. These activities require complex cognitive functions like planning, problem-solving, and fine motor skills. These are essential for maintaining cognitive health and can be particularly valuable for older adults in staving off the signs of mental aging.

Beyond the cognitive benefits, these technology-related hobbies offer a deep sense of accomplishment and fulfillment. Completing a photography project, creating a digital art piece, or publishing a blog post can boost self-esteem and provide a purposeful focus, enriching life in a meaningful way. Therefore, technology-related hobbies are not merely forms of entertainment but potent tools for cognitive engagement and emotional well-being.

Online Courses and Brain Training

The digital landscape is rich with online courses and brain training platforms tailored to suit learners of all ages, including older individuals. These online educational environments offer various subjects, ranging from the sciences and history to arts and crafts, ensuring that there is something to engage almost every interest and passion.

For instance, taking a history course fills gaps in one's knowledge and exercises critical thinking skills. Learners must analyze historical events, evaluate perspectives, and make connections between past and present. Similarly, science courses often involve problem-solving and logic exercises, stimulating different cognitive functions. These courses often come with supplementary materials like quizzes, interactive timelines, or experiments that enrich the learning experience.

Arts and crafts courses provide a different but equally valuable form of cognitive exercise. Learning a new skill, such as painting or knitting, demands creative thinking and fine motor skills. Moreover, such courses often provide opportunities to engage with fellow learners through forums or even virtual classes, thereby adding a social component that can be cognitively beneficial.

Many online platforms also incorporate progress tracking and interactive elements to engage learners. Quizzes, certificates of completion, and forums where students can ask questions and share insights add layers of interactivity that make the learning process more dynamic and rewarding.

But the benefits are not purely cognitive; they also extend to emotional well-being. Achieving milestones in a course or receiving positive feedback can boost self-esteem and provide a sense of accomplishment. Learning itself, especially later in life, can be an empowering experience that instills a renewed sense of purpose.

Cognitive Health Tracking

The rise of apps and wearable devices designed to monitor cognitive health metrics represents a significant advancement in personal health technology. These tools can keep track of various aspects of cognitive function, such as memory, attention span, and reaction time, offering users a more nuanced understanding of their cognitive landscape. It's worth noting that while these devices are not diagnostic tools, they can serve as early warning systems. They can identify trends or irregularities that might warrant further investigation by healthcare professionals. This proactive approach can be invaluable for managing cognitive health effectively.

Moreover, these apps and wearables often come with features that encourage regular cognitive exercise. For instance, they may offer daily brain-training games or mental fitness challenges that prompt users to engage in activities that stimulate cognitive functions. These exercises can serve as practical reminders to take active steps to maintain and improve brain health. The data collected over time can offer insightful patterns and may even be useful for healthcare professionals for a more comprehensive understanding.

However, it's indispensable to be mindful of how technology is used, particularly when it comes to cognitive health. While these devices offer numerous benefits, there is also the risk of becoming overly reliant on them or using them in a way that hampers cognitive function. For example, excessive screen time or the passive consumption of information can have a negative impact. The idea is not to let technology dictate the terms but to incorporate it into a broader, more holistic strategy for maintaining cognitive health.

This means using technology as a supplement rather than a replacement for other proven methods of cognitive maintenance, like physical exercise, social interaction, and a balanced diet. It's also vital to stay updated on the latest research regarding the impact of technology on cognitive health, as this field is continually evolving.

Cognitive Training Interventions

Cognitive training interventions are meticulously designed programs to enhance certain cognitive functions, such as memory retention and problem-solving skills. Unlike generic brain games, these programs are tailored to address an individual's unique cognitive deficits or weaknesses. This customization ensures a targeted approach to achieve specific cognitive goals more effectively.

A variety of engaging techniques are employed in these programs to stimulate cognitive processes. These techniques often include puzzles that challenge logical thinking, memory games that exercise short-term and long-term recall, and even complex tasks that require a combination of cognitive skills. The activities are carefully selected to be not just challenging but also enjoyable, thereby promoting sustained engagement.

The science behind cognitive training interventions relies heavily on the principle of neuroplasticity. Neuroplasticity is the brain's remarkable ability to reorganize by forming new neural connections. This adaptability of the brain allows for the development and strengthening of cognitive skills, even in later stages of life. Through consistent practice, these programs encourage the brain to build new pathways, enhancing its capacity for various mental tasks.

The flexibility of cognitive training interventions allows them to be delivered through different platforms. Some programs are computer-based, leveraging cutting-edge software to engage users in mental exercises. Others are conducted in more traditional settings, such as group or individual sessions led by certified professionals. Regardless of the delivery method, these interventions are evidence-based and grounded in scientific research, demonstrating their effectiveness for a wide range of populations. This includes healthy adults looking to sharpen their mental acuity and individuals dealing with cognitive impairments or recovering from brain injuries.

An indispensable component of successful cognitive training is consistent practice and diligent progress tracking. Continuous engagement and regular assessments allow for fine-tuning interventions, making them increasingly effective over time. In many cases, cognitive training can serve as a complementary therapy, augmenting other medical or psychological treatments an individual may be undergoing.

Given the specialized and personalized nature of cognitive training interventions, consultation with healthcare professionals is usually advised. A thorough evaluation can help determine these programs' suitability and potential effectiveness for an individual's specific cognitive needs and overall health condition. Pursuing mentally stimulating activities and embracing technology as a learning tool can significantly enhance cognitive abilities and support brain health. By challenging your mind, promoting neural connections, and fostering neuroplasticity, you can maintain and improve your cognitive function, contributing to a fulfilling and intellectually vibrant life.

Reflections on The Importance of Continuous Learning

The idea that continuous learning could safeguard against memory loss hits close to home for many of us. Who hasn't worried about forgetting important dates, names, or even broader life memories? The beauty of incorporating continuous learning into our daily lives is that it serves dual purposes: it enriches our world, making each day more interesting, and at the same time, it gives our brains the workout they need to stay sharp.

Let's talk about neuroplasticity—this isn't just a fancy scientific term. It means that our brains have the remarkable ability to adapt and change, no matter our age. When we learn something new—be it a cooking technique, a few phrases in a foreign language, or how to play a musical instrument—we're essentially telling our brain to sit up and take notice, to forge new pathways that make us more resilient to the wear and tear of aging.

But it's not just about tackling massive challenges or becoming an expert in a new field. Simple acts like reading a new genre of literature, engaging in meaningful conversations, or even attending a community class can wake up dormant parts of our brains. And let's not forget that learning can be a social activity, offering the double benefit of emotional connection and cognitive exercise.

Even more exciting is that this approach to cognitive health doesn't have to stand alone. It can easily be integrated with other lifestyle choices to make a comprehensive plan for aging well. Imagine pairing your newfound love for painting with regular physical exercise and a balanced diet. Now, that's a holistic approach to maintaining cognitive health!

Suppose you're considering incorporating more learning into your life to protect your memory. In that case, chatting with your healthcare provider is always a good idea. They can help guide you toward activities that align with your interests and health status, creating a personalized strategy to safeguard your cognitive function and enrich your life immeasurably.

CHAPTER 8

Balancing Stress and Memory

Stress has become an all-too-familiar companion for many of us in a world that often feels like a relentless cycle of responsibilities and deadlines. However, it's important to recognize that while stress is a natural physiological response, its chronic presence can have profound implications for our memory and cognitive function. By shedding light on this complex relationship, we can empower ourselves to make informed choices that promote optimal cognitive health in the face of life's challenges.

In today's fast-paced and demanding world, excessive stress has become a prevalent concern that transcends age, gender, and occupation. While stress is a natural response to challenging situations, its chronic and overwhelming presence can exact a toll on the core of our well-being—the brain. This intricate organ, responsible for cognition, emotions, and our overall mental landscape, is profoundly influenced by the levels of stress we endure.

The following exploration delves into the intricate relationship between excessive stress and brain health. We uncover how prolonged stress can shape the brain's structure, function, and overall cognitive performance. From structural alterations in critical brain regions to disruptions in neurotransmitter balance, we journey into the complex terrain where stress and brain health intersect, ultimately aiming to shed light on the importance of stress management for a resilient and thriving mind.

Cortisol Production

You've probably felt that adrenaline rush when facing a challenge or threat, making your senses sharper and your reactions quicker. This is your body's "fight or flight" response at work, pumping cortisol to help you handle what's right in front of you. In these moments, cortisol is your ally, focusing your attention and giving you that boost of energy to tackle the task at hand.

But what happens when that stress doesn't let up? Maybe it's a demanding job, family issues, or just the relentless pace of modern life. When stress becomes a constant companion, your body keeps

63

churning out cortisol, and that's when things can start to go awry. This hormone, so useful in short bursts, can begin to wear you down over time. Your memory might feel foggy, concentrating becomes harder, and you might even struggle with simple tasks. That's the hippocampus—your brain's memory center—feeling the impact of sustained high cortisol levels.

And it's not just your brain that's affected. You might notice you're not sleeping as well as you used to, or maybe you're gaining weight despite eating the same. Elevated cortisol can throw several aspects of your well-being off balance, from your sleep quality to your heart health.

So, if you're finding that stress has become more of a chronic condition than an acute reaction, it's important to take steps to manage it. Whether that means lifestyle changes like exercise and mindfulness practices or seeking professional guidance for cognitive behavioral therapy or medication, addressing the stress in your life is fundamental to maintaining your cognitive sharpness and overall health.

Realizing the dual role of cortisol as an immediate helper and a long-term challenge is the first step in taking more control over your stress levels and, by extension, your cognitive well-being. Memory Problems

Chronic stress has a notable impact on memory functions. Prolonged exposure to elevated cortisol levels can disrupt the normal functioning of brain regions responsible for memory formation and retrieval. As a result, individuals experiencing chronic stress may struggle to recall and retain new information. This memory impairment can affect daily life, from learning and academic performance to work-related tasks.

Impaired Decision-Making

We've all been there—those times when stress seems to grip our lives, refusing to let go. During these extended periods of stress, we might start noticing something unsettling: our decision-making isn't what it used to be. Our once-sharp ability to evaluate options, weigh potential outcomes, and make well-informed choices has taken a hit.

Chronic stress doesn't just come alone; it often brings along its companions, like heightened anxiety and cognitive rigidity. Imagine trying to solve a puzzle with pieces that don't quite fit together. That's what it can feel like when we're faced with complex decisions under the weight of chronic stress. The mental fog, constant worrying, and feeling stuck in the same thought patterns all conspire against our ability to make clear and effective choices.

The consequences of impaired decision-making can ripple through our lives, affecting personal and professional spheres. It might lead to strained relationships in our personal lives as we struggle to see different perspectives or make compromises. It can hinder our performance at work, making it challenging to navigate complex projects or respond effectively to shifting priorities. Chronic stress can feel like a fog that clouds our judgment, making it difficult to navigate life's intricate maze.

Recognizing this impact on our decision-making is the first step in regaining control over our cognitive well-being. It's a reminder that self-care isn't just a buzzword; it's a practical necessity. Whether through relaxation techniques, seeking support from friends and professionals, or making lifestyle changes to reduce stressors, finding ways to manage chronic stress can help us regain our clarity of thought and ability to make choices that align with our values and goals. Increased Risk of Mental Disorders

Chronic stress is a recognized risk factor for developing mental disorders. Excessive cortisol production, as seen in chronic stress, can negatively impact brain regions responsible for regulating mood. This disruption in mood regulation can contribute to the onset of mental health conditions such as anxiety disorders, depression, and post-traumatic stress disorder (PTSD). Managing stress mitigates the risk of these debilitating mental disorders and promotes overall psychological well-being.

Stress Management Techniques

In today's fast-paced and demanding world, stress has become an inescapable aspect of daily life. Its omnipresence can often leave us feeling overwhelmed and drained, with our mental clarity and emotional stability hanging in the balance. However, possessing the ability to effectively manage stress is a game-changing skill that can protect our brain health, bolster our cognitive function, and fortify our emotional resilience.

The importance of stress management in preserving cognitive function cannot be overstated. Chronic stress can have a detrimental impact on brain health, leading to impaired memory, reduced focus, and decreased cognitive flexibility. It can even contribute to the development of mental health disorders, such as depression and anxiety, further compromising our ability to navigate life's challenges. By mastering effective stress management techniques, we can mitigate these effects, bolstering our brain's resilience and optimizing our cognitive performance.

Stress management encompasses a wide range of strategies, from lifestyle modifications to relaxation techniques. These approaches help to mitigate the physiological and psychological impacts of stress, promoting mental clarity, emotional equilibrium, and overall well-being.

One of the most effective stress management techniques is physical activity. Regular exercise benefits not only physical health but also promotes cognitive function by reducing stress, improving mood, and enhancing sleep quality. Furthermore, exercise stimulates the release of endorphins, the body's natural "feel-good" hormones, which promote relaxation and well-being.

Deep Breathing Exercises

A method that can become your go-to tool for managing stress is deep breathing exercises. Let's take you through your personal experience with this practice. Picture a typical day packed with deadlines, responsibilities, and the unrelenting pace of life. That's when you can pause, finding solace in the rhythmic cadence of your breath. One technique you can often turn to is diaphragmatic breathing, where each breath is a deliberate, intentional act. It's not just inhale-exhale; it's a journey of calm and grounding. As you breathe deeply, you can almost feel the tension in your muscles slowly melting away, like a weight being lifted off your shoulders.

Another technique that can work wonders for you is the 4-7-8 method. It's a simple sequence—inhale for 4 seconds, hold for 7 seconds, and exhale for 8 seconds. It's a systematic process that engages your entire being. Each cycle returns your heart rate to a steady, rhythmic beat, like a calming lullaby for your nervous system. The hold between breaths creates a space—a precious moment of stillness in a world that often feels relentlessly busy.

What's remarkable about these deep breathing exercises is their ability to alleviate stress's mental and physical symptoms. When stress takes hold, it can manifest as muscle tension, a racing heart, or shallow breathing. But with each deep breath, you can feel your muscles relaxing, your heart rate steadying and your breath becoming more profound. It's as if you're telling your body, "It's okay; we're safe." This simple self-care sends a powerful signal to your nervous system, shifting it from a state of alertness to one of calm.

In those moments of deep breathing, you create a sanctuary within yourself—a sanctuary of calm and tranquility that you can return to whenever needed. It's like having a secret weapon against stress, always at your disposal. As you continue to practice these exercises, you can find that their effects linger, creating an undercurrent of serenity that weaves through your day, helping you face challenges with a sense of poise and resilience.

So, from your journey, you can attest to the remarkable power of deep breathing exercises in managing stress. They are not just techniques but lifelines to a place of peace within you, waiting to be discovered and embraced. If you haven't explored these methods yet, take a few moments and breathe deeply. You might find that your well of calm and resilience lies within your breath.

Engaging in Relaxing Activities

Engaging in relaxing activities is an essential strategy for enhancing memory and managing stress. These activities provide a mental and emotional environment where cognitive functions can thrive, making them integral to preserving and improving memory.

Consider reading, for instance. When you lose yourself in a captivating story or delve into the wisdom of a non-fiction book, you allow your brain to explore new horizons. Reading offers a mental break from stressors, stimulates cognitive functions, and enhances memory.

Listening to soothing music is another valuable practice. The gentle melodies and harmonious tunes can transport you to a place of serenity, melting away the tension that accumulates throughout the day. Music's ability to tap into your emotions creates a profound sense of well-being, positively affecting memory and cognitive clarity.

Gardening is a physical and mindful activity that provides a connection with the natural world. Tending to plants, nurturing them, and witnessing their growth creates a sense of calm and invigorates your mind, making remembering and retaining information more accessible.

Artistic pursuits, such as painting or creative writing, offer avenues for self-expression and mental restoration. Engaging in these activities provides an emotional outlet and encourages cognitive flexibility and imagination, both vital aspects of memory.

These relaxing activities create a conducive environment for cognitive well-being, making them necessary for maintaining and enhancing memory. Whether through reading, music, gardening, or creative endeavors, these moments of tranquility can be profound investments in your cognitive health.

Mindfulness Meditation

Mindfulness meditation is like a soothing balm for the chaos of our modern lives. It's a practice that is incredibly valuable in navigating the turbulent waters of stress. Mindfulness meditation is about intentionally bringing your focus to the here and now, allowing you to acknowledge and accept your thoughts and feelings without judgment.

Imagine this scenario: deadlines are looming, emails are piling up, and life's endless demands seem overwhelming. That's when mindfulness meditation steps in as your steadfast ally. It encourages you to pause, find a quiet corner, and be present. It's not about denying your feelings or pushing thoughts away; it's about observing them, recognizing them for what they are, and letting them pass through your mind like clouds drifting across the sky.

What's remarkable is how this practice can profoundly impact your stress levels. Through mindfulness, you cultivate a deep sense of relaxation. It's as if you're gently turning down the volume on the cacophony of daily life, finding a calm center within yourself. Sitting with your thoughts and feelings without the constant urge to react allows you to regain control in the face of life's challenges.

Moreover, mindfulness meditation is like a master class in emotional regulation. It's a skill that I've honed over time, and it has helped me navigate the rollercoaster of emotions that often accompany stress. Instead of being swept away by anger, frustration, or anxiety, you learn to observe these emotions with curiosity and compassion. This process allows you to respond to them more balanced and measuredly rather than impulsively.

Perhaps one of the most transformative aspects of mindfulness is its power to increase self-awareness. It's like holding up a mirror to your inner world, getting to know yourself deeper. Through this self-awareness, you recognize your habitual thought patterns and reactions, which can be enlightening and empowering.

Regular mindfulness meditation, woven into the fabric of daily life, can rewire your brain's response to stressors. It's not about eliminating stress; that's an impossible task in our complex world. Instead, it's about becoming more resilient in the face of stress, approaching challenges calmly and composedly.

Social Support

The profound influence of human connection as a potent antidote to stress cannot be overstated. In the intricate web of our lives, the bonds we share with friends, family members, and even mental health professionals serve as invaluable shields against stress. When life's challenges seem insurmountable, reaching out to these trusted individuals can provide a key buffer, nurturing our mental well-being and emotional fortitude.

Picture a moment when stress feels like an ever-encroaching shadow, threatening to cast a pall over your daily existence. Talking about your stressors takes on a remarkable significance in these moments. A profound transformation begins as you unburden yourself, sharing your thoughts, worries, and feelings with someone you trust. It's as if verbalizing these concerns is like opening a release valve, allowing the pent-up emotional pressure to escape. The weight on your shoulders begins to lift, and the emotional burdens that stress brings dissipate.

This process is further illuminated by the empathetic and wise guidance of those you turn to. Whether it's a close friend who understands your journey, a family member who has witnessed your trials and triumphs, or a mental health professional equipped with the tools to navigate the complexities of stress, their support is like a lifeline in turbulent waters. Their empathy and advice offer more than just words; they are a beacon of hope and solace.

In these moments, human connection doesn't merely alleviate emotional burdens; it also fosters resilience. Through the shared experiences, the listening ear, and the supportive embrace, you come to realize that you are not alone in facing life's challenges. This knowledge is like a cornerstone upon which emotional fortitude is built. It provides the strength to weather the storms of life, knowing that you have a network of support to fall back on.

Human connection isn't just a remedy for stress; it's a vital source of emotional and mental sustenance. It's a testament to the profound impact that our relationships with others can have on our overall well-being. Thus, from these reflections, we can affirm the enduring truth that sharing our stressors, expressing our feelings, and seeking support from trusted individuals are not signs of weakness but powerful strategies for maintaining emotional equilibrium and emerging from the trials of life with greater resilience and strength.

Reflections on Balancing Stress and Memory

Building stress resilience emerges as a proactive and empowering strategy for effectively managing the constant ebb and flow of life's challenges. Think of it as assembling a robust strategy toolkit that empowers you to navigate the often-turbulent waters of stress with grace and composure. The profound impact of excessive stress on our lives cannot be underestimated, as its repercussions extend into various facets of our well-being.

One area where stress has a significant influence is brain health. The brain, our command center for cognitive functions and emotional well-being, is particularly susceptible to the corrosive effects of unmanaged stress. It's not uncommon for chronic stress to manifest as tangible issues like memory problems, difficulties in making sound decisions, and an elevated vulnerability to mental health disorders. Under the prolonged duress of unmitigated stress, the brain can undergo wear and tear that diminishes its cognitive functions and overall resilience.

However, amidst this landscape of potential adversity, there's a gleaming silver lining in stress management. By seamlessly incorporating a diverse range of effective stress management approaches into your daily routine, you are taking proactive steps to counteract the negative impacts of stress.

This journey of building stress resilience is akin to a path of self-discovery and empowerment. It equips you with a toolbox full of strategies that mitigate the deleterious effects of stress and contribute to a healthier, more resilient brain and mind.

It's a vital endeavor that nurtures a resilient mind capable of confronting life's challenges head-on, ultimately leading to a richer and more fulfilling life.

CHAPTER 9

Managing Depression for A Better Memory

Exploring the realm of depression reveals its deep influence, extending beyond mere mood to vital cognitive processes like memory and attention. Despite facing formidable challenges, there is hope in strategies designed to address depression's impact. By embracing lifestyle changes, individuals can meticulously safeguard their cognitive well-being, regaining control over their mental faculties.

Depression is a multifaceted and frequently debilitating mental health condition that reaches far beyond its immediate effects on mood and emotional well-being. Its far-reaching influence extends to the core of cognitive processes, where it can profoundly impact Important aspects like memory and attention. These cognitive functions are the building blocks of our daily lives, shaping our ability to engage with the world and navigate its complexities. However, when depression sets in, it's as though a shadow descends upon these mental processes, affecting them in intricate ways.

Understanding the intricate relationship between depression and the brain's structure and neurotransmitter balance is essential to comprehend this condition. Depression's impact on cognitive function is intertwined with these underlying neurological factors. Yet, even in the face of such formidable challenges, there is hope and empowerment. By delving into strategies to address depression's cognitive impact, we can unlock the potential for improvement.

Embarking on this comprehensive journey towards cognitive restoration in the face of depression may seem daunting at first, but each step forward signifies progress. Each lifestyle change, each healthy habit, each connection made, and each mindful moment contributes a piece to the mosaic of cognitive restoration, illuminating a path toward a brighter and more empowered future. By embracing this holistic approach, individuals can regain control over their cognitive faculties and reshape their mental landscape, banishing the shadows of depression and fostering a renewed sense of hope and optimism for the future.

How Depression Affects Memory

When depression takes hold, it often brings a host of cognitive challenges. Memory, which encompasses information encoding, storage, and retrieval, can become notably impaired. Individuals with depression often report difficulties remembering everyday tasks, recalling recent conversations, or focusing on routine activities.

This cognitive fog can be frustrating and can further deepen the emotional burden of depression. Additionally, depression tends to shorten attention spans, making concentrating on tasks and absorbing new information harder. Understanding these cognitive effects is imperative in providing comprehensive support and intervention for those grappling with depression, as it highlights the interconnectedness of mental health and cognitive well-being.

Impaired Concentration

When depression takes hold, you may grapple with a profound challenge that affects many aspects of your daily life: maintaining focus. Whether you're at work, attempting to study, or simply going about your routine tasks, depression can cast a dense cloud over your ability to concentrate. It's as if this emotional weight envelops your mind, creating a thick fog that makes it significantly more difficult to encode new information effectively into memory.

In these moments, it can be incredibly frustrating. The already complex emotional landscape of depression is further complicated by the struggle to retain and recall essential details. It's as though you're navigating a maze with an extra layer of barriers, each one making it harder to see the path forward.

Reduced Attention Span

Enduring the persistent weight of melancholy or indifference that often accompanies depression is akin to carrying a heavy burden day in and day out. This emotional load profoundly affects your attention span, affecting your ability to focus and engage with the world around you. It's as though there's a constant struggle to maintain concentration, and this internal battle becomes increasingly draining over time.

Consequently, you may find that your capacity to sustain attention wanes, making it challenging to immerse yourself in tasks

72

or conversations fully. Mundane activities that were once straightforward can become Herculean feats. Even something as seemingly routine as reading a book or following a conversation can feel like an uphill climb.

The compromise in your ability to concentrate isn't limited to the present moment; it extends its grasp into your memory. With your attention span diminished, the brain's capacity to absorb and retain new information is significantly impacted. This, in turn, can lead to difficulties in recalling details, events, or facts that were once well within your grasp. The metaphor of depression as a formidable barrier is apt. It's as though your mind is enclosed within a fortress, limiting its receptivity to new knowledge and experiences. This can be incredibly frustrating as opportunities for personal growth and learning are slipping away.

Negative Cognitive Bias

One of the hallmark features of depression is the presence of a negative cognitive bias. This bias operates as a mental filter, causing individuals to disproportionately focus on and remember adverse events and emotions while concurrently downplaying or even overlooking positive ones. This skewed perspective can have a profound impact on how individuals perceive and interpret their experiences, and it carries a significant influence over how they recall memories.

Imagine it as a lens through which life is viewed, one that tends to magnify the shadows and dim the light. For someone grappling with depression, they may vividly remember failures, setbacks, or painful experiences with remarkable clarity. These memories can become like indelible imprints on the mind, often haunting their thoughts. In contrast, moments of joy, success, or happiness may seem fleeting and elusive, slipping away from memory like grains of sand through their fingers.

This cognitive bias holds immense power. It reinforces the feelings of sadness and despair that often accompany depression, creating a reinforcing loop where negative thoughts and emotions seem to confirm their bleak outlook. Additionally, it compounds the impact on memory function, making it even more challenging to recall positive experiences or aspects of life that could provide solace and hope.

Hippocampal Atrophy

Chronic depression takes a toll not only on one's emotional well-being but also on the very structure of the brain, particularly the hippocampus, a region pivotal for memory functions. This intricate relationship between depression and the brain's architecture becomes evident over time. Prolonged exposure to the stress hormones that often accompany depression can lead to significant structural changes, notably the phenomenon known as hippocampal atrophy.

Hippocampal atrophy is a process where this vital brain region gradually shrinks in size. This transformation has profound consequences, especially in the realm of memory. As the hippocampus deteriorates, its once-efficient ability to process and store new information becomes increasingly compromised. This structural change significantly contributes to the memory deficits observed in individuals struggling with depression.

Imagine it as a library that's slowly losing its shelves and capacity to store books. The books represent memories in this analogy, and the shrinking library signifies the diminishing hippocampus. As the shelves disappear, it becomes more challenging to organize, access, and retrieve the stored information accurately.

These memory-related challenges become a part of the complex landscape of chronic depression, adding to individuals' emotional burden. Difficulty retaining and retrieving important information can affect various aspects of daily life, from work to personal relationships.

Strategies to Improve Memory Despite Depression

In the challenging landscape of depression, where cognitive functions like memory often bear the brunt of the disorder, the quest for strategies to improve memory becomes paramount. Depression's impact on memory is well-documented, but it's not an insurmountable hurdle. Addressing memory issues associated with depression involves a multifaceted approach. Here's an in-depth look at effective strategies to improve memory while managing depression:

1. Seek Treatment

The cornerstone of memory improvement when dealing with depression lies in addressing the depression itself. Depression casts a long shadow over various aspects of life, including cognitive function, memory, and overall well-being. It's like a heavy cloud that obscures the sun, making it challenging to see clearly and remember effectively.

74

One of the most effective approaches to tackling depression is engaging in therapy, particularly cognitive-behavioral therapy (CBT). CBT is a structured and evidence-based form of therapy that helps individuals identify and challenge negative thought patterns and behaviors. Through CBT, individuals can gain valuable insights into their thought processes, learn healthier ways to cope with stress and negative emotions and develop more adaptive strategies for managing life's challenges.

In some cases, medication prescribed by a healthcare professional may also be a valuable tool in alleviating depressive symptoms. Medications can help restore the balance of neurotransmitters in the brain, significantly regulating mood and cognitive function. This restoration of balance can lead to improvements in memory and other cognitive processes.

It's important to emphasize that the decision to pursue therapy or medication should be made in consultation with a healthcare professional who can provide personalized guidance based on an individual's unique circumstances and needs. These professionals can assess the severity of depression, consider any coexisting conditions, and tailor a treatment plan that addresses both depressive symptoms and cognitive challenges.

Ultimately, by taking steps to address depression through therapy and, when appropriate, medication, individuals can experience relief from the emotional burden of depression and, in turn, find improvement in their cognitive abilities, including memory. It's a journey toward better mental health and enhanced overall well-being, where the clouds of depression gradually part, allowing the brightness of memory and cognitive vitality to shine through once more.

2. Exercise Regularly

Physical activity's profound impact on mood and cognitive function cannot be overstated. Engaging in regular exercise has been shown to be a powerful tool in promoting not only physical health but also mental well-being.

When you exercise, your body responds by releasing a cascade of chemicals and neurotransmitters that play key roles in mood regulation and memory enhancement. Two of the most notable neurotransmitters in this regard are serotonin and dopamine. Serotonin is often called the "feel-good" neurotransmitter because it contributes to a sense of well-being and happiness. On the other hand, dopamine is involved in reward-motivated behavior and plays an important role in motivation and pleasure.

By releasing these neurotransmitters, exercise can remarkably elevate mood, reduce stress and anxiety, and enhance overall emotional well-being. This mood improvement can have a direct positive impact on memory and cognitive function. When you're feeling happier and less stressed, your brain is better equipped to focus, process information, and store memories effectively.

Incorporating physical activity into your routine, whether through regular workouts, walking, swimming, or engaging in sports, can thus be seen as a valuable memory-enhancing tool. It's like giving your brain a natural and invigorating boost, improving its ability to function optimally.

Furthermore, exercise has been linked to the growth and preservation of brain cells, particularly in regions responsible for memory, such as the hippocampus. This neuroplasticity, or the brain's ability to adapt and change, is stimulated by physical activity, further reinforcing the notion that exercise is good for both the body and the mind.

So, whether you're looking to boost your mood, reduce stress, or enhance your memory, incorporating regular physical activity into your life is a holistic approach that offers numerous benefits. It's a way to nurture your physical and mental well-being, helping you lead a happier, more fulfilling life while promoting optimal cognitive function and memory.

3. Healthy Diet

A healthy diet can significantly impact the management and prevention of depression. Nutrition, while not a sole remedy for clinical depression, can be a valuable complement to other treatments, fostering improved mental well-being. A balanced diet provides essential nutrients supporting brain function, such as omega-3 fatty acids, B vitamins, and antioxidants. These nutrients play vital roles in mood regulation and overall mental health. Foods rich in these nutrients, such as fatty fish, leafy greens, and whole grains, can be beneficial.

Emerging research highlights the connection between the gut and the brain, known as the gut-brain axis. A diet rich in fiber, probiotics, and prebiotics helps maintain a healthy gut microbiome, potentially impacting mood and reducing depression risk.

Managing blood sugar levels is another facet. Diets high in refined sugars and processed foods lead to blood sugar fluctuations, affecting mood and energy levels and potentially contributing to depressive symptoms. Eating complex carbohydrates, fiber-rich foods, and balanced meals helps stabilize blood sugar.

Chronic inflammation is linked to mood disorders, including depression. An anti-inflammatory diet, including fatty fish, nuts, and colorful fruits and vegetables, can reduce inflammation and potentially alleviate depressive symptoms. Hydration is often overlooked; dehydration can affect mood and cognitive function, so staying well-hydrated is essential.

Additionally, moderating or avoiding substances like caffeine and alcohol can be key for individuals prone to depression, as both can disrupt sleep patterns and exacerbate mood swings.

It's vital to recognize that dietary changes alone may not suffice for severe depression. Seek professional help from mental health providers when experiencing depression. However, incorporating a healthy diet into an overall wellness strategy can complement treatments and improve mood and mental well-being. Managing depression involves multiple factors, including physical activity, sleep, stress management, social support, and, when necessary, professional guidance.

4. Quality Sleep

Quality sleep plays a pivotal role in the management and impact of depression. Depression often disrupts sleep patterns and sleep disturbances can exacerbate depressive symptoms. The relationship between depression and sleep is complex, but understanding how they influence each other is Important for effective management.

Sleep disturbances are common in depression, leading to difficulty falling asleep, waking up too early, or experiencing restless, non-restorative sleep. These problems can intensify feelings of fatigue, sadness, and hopelessness, worsening the overall experience of depression.

Moreover, poor sleep quality or insufficient sleep can profoundly affect mood regulation, resulting in increased irritability, mood swings, and heightened emotional reactivity—all of which can further exacerbate depressive symptoms.

In addition to mood-related consequences, sleep is essential for memory consolidation and cognitive function. Disrupted sleep patterns in depression can impair memory recall, decision-making, and problem-solving abilities, adding to the cognitive challenges individuals with depression may face.

The relationship between sleep and depression often forms a vicious cycle, with depression leading to sleep disturbances and those disturbances, in turn, exacerbating depressive symptoms.

Breaking this cycle often requires addressing the underlying depression and implementing effective sleep hygiene practices.

Addressing sleep disturbances is an indispensable aspect of managing depression effectively. Healthcare professionals may recommend therapies focusing on improving sleep quality, such as cognitive-behavioral therapy for insomnia (CBT-I). Additionally, medications prescribed for depression can influence sleep patterns, and healthcare providers may adjust medication regimens to mitigate sleep-related side effects.

Practicing good sleep hygiene is vital for individuals with depression. Establishing a regular sleep schedule, creating a comfortable sleep environment, and limiting screen time before bed are some strategies that can help improve sleep quality. By prioritizing quality sleep, individuals with depression can enhance their mood and cognitive function, contributing to a better overall quality of life.

5. Stay Socially Active

Maintaining an active social life can significantly impact managing and coping with depression. Depression often leads to social withdrawal and isolation, further exacerbating the condition. Engaging in social activities provides opportunities for meaningful human connections, reducing loneliness and fostering a sense of belonging. These interactions can offer emotional support, validation, and a sense of understanding, helping to alleviate depressive symptoms. Social activities also distract from negative thoughts and rumination, providing moments of respite from the emotional burdens of depression.

Additionally, they can boost self-esteem and self-worth, counteracting the negative self-perceptions often associated with depression. Regular physical activity, often a component of social activities, has mood-lifting effects and can be beneficial for managing depression. Social commitments provide structure and routine, which can be especially helpful when depression disrupts daily life. By fostering meaningful social connections and openly discussing their experiences, individuals with depression can find valuable sources of emotional support, understanding, and encouragement on their journey toward better mental health.

6. Cognitive Training

Cognitive training exercises offer a valuable tool for individuals with depression to sharpen their memory and overall cognitive abilities. These activities, such as puzzles, memory games, and learning new skills, engage the brain and promote mental agility. Depression often brings cognitive challenges, including difficulties with concentration and memory recall. Cognitive training exercises can help combat these issues by stimulating the brain's neural pathways. Puzzles and memory games, for example, require focused attention and problem-solving skills, enhancing concentration and memory retention.

Learning new skills or acquiring knowledge in different areas provides mental stimulation and a sense of accomplishment and self-esteem, which can be particularly important for individuals dealing with the emotional weight of depression.

Cognitive training exercises can also be a constructive and enjoyable way to fill one's time, offering a sense of purpose and achievement. It's important to note that cognitive training exercises should be part of a holistic approach to managing depression, which may include therapy and, in some cases, medication.

7. Keep a Journal

Writing down your thoughts, experiences, and emotions can be a therapeutic outlet and aid in memory recall. Maintaining a journal can offer several benefits for individuals dealing with depression.

Firstly, writing provides an emotional release valve, allowing you to express your feelings in a safe and private space, relieving the emotional burdens associated with depression. Secondly, journaling enhances memory recall by documenting experiences and thoughts, which can be especially valuable when depression affects cognitive function, making it difficult to remember important details.

Additionally, regular journaling enables you to track mood changes over time, offering insights into the patterns and triggers of depressive episodes, which can help you and your mental health professional develop effective coping strategies.

Moreover, writing allows for self-reflection, helping you better understand your thoughts and emotions and identify negative thought patterns to work towards more positive and constructive thinking. Maintaining a journal can help you set and track personal goals, providing a sense of accomplishment and motivation, which is critical for individuals with depression.

Your journal becomes a record of your journey through depression, documenting both the challenges and the triumphs, serving as a source of inspiration and resilience over time, showcasing how you've overcome obstacles and grown.

Lastly, journaling can facilitate communication with mental health professionals, providing valuable insights into your experiences and making it easier to tailor your treatment plan. Whether through traditional pen-and-paper journaling or digital platforms, writing down your thoughts and experiences can be a therapeutic tool for managing depression and enhancing memory recall.

8. Manage Stress

Stress management techniques play a pivotal role in mitigating memory problems associated with depression. Methods like deep breathing exercises, progressive muscle relaxation, and effective time management are instrumental in reducing stress levels, which can significantly enhance cognitive function.

Deep breathing exercises promote relaxation by engaging the body's relaxation response. Techniques like diaphragmatic breathing or the 4-7-8 method (inhale for 4 seconds, hold for 7 seconds, exhale for 8 seconds) involve slow, deliberate breaths that can alleviate physical symptoms of stress, such as muscle tension and an increased heart rate. This, in turn, contributes to a state of calm, reducing the cognitive load imposed by stress.

Progressive muscle relaxation, another valuable technique, involves systematically tensing and relaxing different muscle groups in the body. This not only helps release physical tension but also promotes mental relaxation. As stress often manifests in physical symptoms, addressing both the body and mind can benefit memory and overall cognitive function.

Effective time management is also imperative in reducing stress. It allows individuals to prioritize tasks, allocate sufficient time for each, and avoid the overwhelming feeling of being constantly rushed or burdened by an unmanageable workload. By creating a structured routine, individuals can minimize the mental strain caused by disorganization and time-related stressors, creating a more conducive environment for memory and cognitive function.

Overall, these stress management techniques provide individuals with practical tools to navigate the challenges of depression and its impact on memory. By incorporating them into their daily lives, individuals can work towards reducing stress-related memory problems and ultimately enhancing their cognitive well-being.

The key takeaway is that stress management techniques like deep breathing exercises, progressive muscle relaxation, and effective time management are instrumental in mitigating memory

80

problems associated with depression. These techniques help reduce stress levels, which can significantly enhance cognitive function and alleviate the negative impact of depression on memory.

9. Practice Mindfulness

Practicing mindfulness can be a transformative strategy for individuals dealing with depression, especially when it comes to managing its effects on cognitive function, including memory. Mindfulness entails intentionally focusing on the present moment while acknowledging and accepting one's thoughts and emotions without judgment. This technique has been shown to reduce stress by promoting relaxation, enhancing emotional regulation, and increasing self-awareness.

For those struggling with depression, mindfulness offers several tangible benefits. Firstly, it can significantly reduce stress, an everyday companion of depression, by helping individuals manage and alleviate it. By learning to stay present and not dwell on past regrets or future worries, individuals often experience a greater sense of calm and emotional balance.

Secondly, mindfulness practices facilitate emotional regulation, which can be particularly valuable when depression leads to intense and overwhelming emotions. It encourages individuals to observe their emotions without judgment, providing a healthier response to challenging feelings. This can help individuals gain better control over their emotional responses and reduce the emotional toll that depression can have on memory. Mindfulness fosters self-awareness by encouraging individuals to pay close attention to their thoughts and feelings. This heightened self-awareness enables them to identify negative thought patterns and triggers for depressive episodes, empowering them to address these issues effectively.

Moreover, engaging in mindfulness exercises can lead to enhanced cognitive function, including memory. By training the mind to focus on the present moment, individuals can improve their ability to concentrate and remember important details, which can be particularly valuable when depression affects cognitive function.

Lastly, regular mindfulness practice can rewire the brain to respond to stressors more calmly and resiliently. This can reduce the impact of depression on memory and cognitive function, contributing to better overall mental well-being.

While mindfulness is not a standalone solution for depression, it can be a valuable complementary approach to therapy and medication. By incorporating mindfulness into their daily routine, individuals can work towards managing the effects of depression on memory and enhancing their overall cognitive health.

10. Consult a Professional

Suppose memory issues persist or worsen despite dedicated efforts to manage depression. In that case, seeking guidance from a neuropsychologist or a healthcare professional with expertise in cognitive assessments is advisable. These specialists can offer tailored strategies and recommendations to address memory challenges effectively, considering each individual's unique circumstances.

It's important to remember that recovery from depression is a gradual process. As depressive symptoms subside through therapy, medication, and lifestyle changes, memory and cognitive function improvements often follow suit. Being patient with oneself and recognizing that progress may take time is Important for achieving better memory and overall well-being.

In summary, if memory problems continue to be a concern despite managing depression, consulting a qualified healthcare professional can provide valuable insights and solutions. Remember that seeking support and being patient with the process are essential to improved memory and cognitive health.

Reflections on Managing Depression for a Better Memory

Depression, a mental health condition characterized by persistent feelings of sadness and hopelessness, is often associated with emotional distress and mood disturbances. However, its impact extends beyond the emotional realm, reaching into the depths of cognitive function. Understanding the intricate ways in which depression can affect memory, attention, and cognitive biases is key to fostering empathy and guiding effective treatment strategies.

One of the key areas where depression's impact is felt is memory. Individuals experiencing depression may struggle with memory retrieval and recall, often finding it challenging to remember specific events or details. This impairment in memory can be attributed to depression-related changes in brain chemistry and structure, including alterations in the hippocampus, a region essential for memory formation.

Depression's reach also extends to attention and concentration. Individuals grappling with this mental health condition may find it challenging to focus on tasks, resulting in a shortened attention span. This diminished concentration can have far-reaching implications, affecting productivity, academic performance, and overall cognitive function. The inability to concentrate can exacerbate feelings of frustration and inadequacy, further perpetuating the cycle of depression.

Amid this intricate and challenging terrain, understanding the effects of depression on cognitive function is invaluable. It fosters a deeper sense of empathy and guides the development of personalized treatment strategies that address the multifaceted nature of this mental health condition.

Depression's impact extends beyond emotional distress, permeating the intricate domains of cognitive function. By understanding the diverse ways in which memory, attention, and cognitive biases can be affected by depression, we gain valuable insights for fostering empathy, guiding treatment, and empowering individuals to navigate the challenges that arise.

CHAPTER 10

Medications and Memory Interactions

Taking medication isn't just about fixing what's physically or emotionally wrong—it's a pact with your brain. Some meds can boost your memory and focus, while others might make you foggy or forgetful. Awareness of these changes isn't just good healthcare; it's a deeply personal act of looking after your mind. So, as you manage your meds, remember you're also managing your mental well-being.

The impact of medications on memory and cognitive well-being is of immense significance in healthcare and neurology. Medications, whether prescribed to manage physical health conditions or address mental health concerns, can profoundly influence an individual's cognitive faculties, including memory, attention, and overall cognitive function.

This influence can manifest in various ways, from beneficial effects that enhance cognitive performance to side effects that detrimentally affect memory and mental clarity. Understanding the complex interplay between medications and cognitive well-being is essential for healthcare providers and individuals seeking to make informed choices about their treatment regimens. Medications and cognitive function have a multifaceted relationship.

Medications can significantly impact cognitive function, and understanding their effects is indispensable for maintaining and enhancing memory and overall cognitive abilities. Let's examine the diverse array of drugs that can impact memory and cognition and suggest strategies to optimize cognitive health in the presence of medication-related challenges. Here's an in-depth exploration of how different types of medications can influence cognitive function:

Medications for Cognitive Enhancement

Certain medications, often called nootropics or cognitive enhancers, have gained attention for their ability to enhance cognitive functions, including memory, attention, and concentration. While these drugs are frequently used to address specific medical conditions such as attention deficit hyperactivity disorder (ADHD) or cognitive impairments associated with neurodegenerative diseases like Alzheimer's, they have also piqued the interest of individuals seeking cognitive enhancement.

These medications target neurotransmitters and brain chemicals to improve cognitive performance. For example, some drugs enhance the release of neurotransmitters like dopamine, which is important for memory and focus. Others may modulate brainwave patterns, fostering a state of heightened alertness and cognitive acuity.

It's important to note that the efficacy of these drugs can vary from person to person. While some individuals may experience significant cognitive improvements, others may not respond as strongly or encounter side effects. Furthermore, the long-term safety and potential risks associated with these drugs are still being studied, emphasizing the importance of using them under the guidance of a healthcare professional.

For those who genuinely require these medications to manage specific medical conditions, they can provide profound relief and improvements in cognitive function. However, for individuals seeking cognitive enhancement without a medical necessity, it's essential to approach these drugs cautiously and engage in thorough research while considering potential risks and benefits. Consulting a healthcare professional is advisable to make informed decisions regarding their use.

Psychotropic Medications

Medications prescribed to manage mental health conditions, including antidepressants, antipsychotics, and anxiolytics, can affect cognitive function. Recognizing that the impact of these drugs can vary widely from one individual to another, as well as depending on the specific medication being used.

1. ***Antidepressants:*** Antidepressants are commonly used to treat mood disorders like depression and anxiety. Some individuals report improved cognitive function and memory while taking these medications. This may be due to alleviating symptoms like persistent sadness or anxiety, which can cloud cognitive processes. However, it's important to note that not all antidepressants have the same effects, and some individuals may experience side effects like drowsiness or memory problems.

2. *Antipsychotics:* Antipsychotic medications are primarily used to manage conditions like schizophrenia and bipolar disorder. Their impact on cognition can vary significantly. While they can help reduce symptoms like hallucinations and delusions, some antipsychotics may lead to cognitive blunting or mild memory issues in certain individuals.

3. *Anxiolytics:* Anxiolytics, or anti-anxiety medications, are prescribed to alleviate symptoms of anxiety disorders. These drugs can have varying effects on cognitive function. Some may help improve concentration and memory by reducing excessive worry and anxiety, while others can induce drowsiness or mild cognitive impairment.

Individual response to these medications is key. What works well for one person may not be suitable for another. When prescribing these drugs, healthcare professionals carefully consider an individual's symptoms, medical history, and potential side effects. Suppose someone experiences cognitive side effects that affect their daily functioning. In that case, it's essential to communicate these concerns with their healthcare provider. Adjustments to the medication regimen or exploring alternative treatments may be considered to optimize cognitive well-being while managing mental health conditions effectively.

Sedative-Hypnotic Medications

Sedative-hypnotic drugs, including benzodiazepines commonly prescribed for anxiety and sleep disorders, are known to have potential cognitive side effects, especially when used over extended periods. These medications, while effective in managing symptoms of anxiety and sleep disturbances, can bring about a range of cognitive challenges.

1. *Mental Fog:* Prolonged use of benzodiazepines can lead to a state often described as "mental fog." This refers to a feeling of haziness, where thinking clearly, concentrating, or remembering information becomes challenging. This mental fog can significantly impact daily functioning.

2. *Reduced Cognitive Clarity:* Individuals taking these medications may notice reduced cognitive clarity. This can manifest as difficulties in making decisions, solving problems, or processing information efficiently.

3. *Memory Impairment:* One of the notable cognitive effects of benzodiazepines is memory impairment. Individuals may experience short-term and long-term

86

memory difficulties, making recalling recent events or information challenging.

It's important to note that these cognitive effects can vary from person to person, and not everyone will experience them to the same extent. Additionally, the severity of these effects can be influenced by factors like the dosage, duration of use, and individual sensitivity to the medication.

Due to these potential cognitive side effects, healthcare providers typically consider the risks and benefits of benzodiazepine use when prescribing them. They may explore alternative treatments or therapies for managing anxiety and sleep disorders, particularly in cases where cognitive clarity and memory preservation are crucial. Suppose someone is experiencing cognitive challenges while taking benzodiazepines. In that case, it's essential to communicate these concerns with their healthcare provider for appropriate evaluation and potential adjustments to their treatment plan.

Anticholinergic Medications

Certain medications, including those prescribed for allergies, motion sickness, and overactive bladder, have anticholinergic properties. These drugs work by blocking the action of the neurotransmitter acetylcholine, which plays an imperative role in cognitive function. While these medications can be effective for managing specific conditions, their prolonged use has been associated with potential cognitive side effects, notably memory impairment. This has raised concerns within the medical community about the possibility of an increased risk of dementia associated with long-term use of anticholinergic drugs.

- *Memory Impairment:* The primary cognitive effect of anticholinergic medications is memory impairment. Individuals taking these drugs may experience short-term and long-term memory difficulties, making recalling recent events or information challenging. This can have a noticeable impact on daily functioning and quality of life.
- *Concerns About Dementia:* The cumulative use of anticholinergic medications has prompted concerns about their potential role in increasing the risk of dementia. While the exact relationship between anticholinergic drugs and dementia is complex and not fully understood, research has

suggested a possible link, especially with prolonged and high-dose use.

- **Individual Variation:** It's essential to note that not everyone who takes anticholinergic medications will experience memory impairment or an increased risk of dementia. The severity of these cognitive effects can vary from person to person and may be influenced by factors such as the specific medication, dosage, duration of use, and individual susceptibility.

Given these concerns, healthcare providers carefully consider the risks and benefits of prescribing anticholinergic medications, particularly for older adults and individuals at higher risk of cognitive decline. They may explore alternative treatment options or adjust medication regimens to minimize potential cognitive side effects. It's important for individuals taking these medications to communicate any cognitive concerns with their healthcare provider, as monitoring and adjustments to the treatment plan may be necessary to ensure optimal cognitive function and overall well-being.

Cardiovascular Medications

Certain medications prescribed for cardiovascular conditions, such as beta-blockers, have been associated with potential cognitive effects. It's important to note that the impact on cognition can vary from person to person and may depend on factors like specific medication, dosage, and individual health conditions.

- *Cognitive Impairment:* Some individuals taking beta-blockers have reported experiencing cognitive impairment. This may manifest as difficulties with memory, concentration, or mental clarity. It's essential for individuals taking these medications to be aware of potential cognitive side effects and communicate any concerns with their healthcare provider.
- *Depression:* Besides cognitive effects, beta-blockers have also been linked to depressive symptoms in some individuals. Depression can further impact cognitive function, leading to memory, attention, and decision-making difficulties.
- *Individual Variation:* Not everyone who takes beta-blockers will experience cognitive impairment or depressive symptoms. The response to these medications can vary

88

widely among individuals. Factors such as the specific beta-blocker used, the dosage, and the presence of other health conditions can influence the likelihood and severity of cognitive side effects.

- *Monitoring and Adjustments:* Healthcare providers closely monitor patients when prescribing beta-blockers or similar medications. If cognitive impairment or depressive symptoms are observed, adjustments to the treatment plan may be considered. This could involve modifying the medication dosage, exploring alternative treatments, or addressing underlying factors contributing to cognitive issues.

While beta-blockers and similar cardiovascular medications can have cognitive effects, their impact varies among individuals. Patients must communicate openly with their healthcare providers, report any cognitive concerns, and work collaboratively to optimize cardiovascular health and cognitive function. Adjustments to the treatment plan may be necessary to balance the benefits of these medications with their potential cognitive side effects.

Anti-Seizure Medications
Anti-seizure medications, while indispensable for managing seizures and epilepsy, can indeed have cognitive effects, including impacts on memory. It's important to recognize that the extent and nature of these cognitive effects can vary widely among different medications and individuals. Here are some key points to consider:

1. *Medication Variability:* Several anti-seizure drugs are available, and each may uniquely impact cognitive function. Some medications may be more likely to affect memory and other cognitive processes, while others may have milder or different cognitive side effects.

2. *Individual Response:* The response to anti-seizure drugs can be highly individual. Some individuals may experience noticeable cognitive changes, including memory difficulties, while others may have minimal or no cognitive side effects.

3. *Dosage and Treatment Plan:* Anti-seizure medication dosage and treatment plan can also influence cognitive effects. Adjustments to medication dosages or the addition of complementary therapies may help manage cognitive side effects in some cases.

4. *Balancing Benefits and Risks:* When managing seizures and epilepsy, healthcare providers aim to strike a balance between controlling seizures effectively and minimizing cognitive side effects. In some situations, the choice of medication may be guided by the individual's cognitive needs and tolerability.

5. *Open Communication:* It's key for individuals taking anti-seizure drugs to maintain open communication with their healthcare provider. If they notice changes in memory or other cognitive functions, discussing these concerns with their provider is essential. This allows for adjustments to the treatment plan or consideration of alternative medications.

Anti-seizure medications can indeed affect cognitive function, including memory, but the impact varies among medications and individuals. When managing seizures, individuals need to work closely with their healthcare provider to find the most suitable medication and treatment plan that balances seizure control with cognitive well-being. Regular communication and monitoring can help address any cognitive side effects effectively.

Pain Medications

Opioid pain medications have long been a staple in the management of severe pain, providing much-needed relief for countless individuals dealing with acute and chronic conditions. However, as valuable as these medications can be, there is a growing concern surrounding their potential impact on cognitive function, particularly at higher doses and with prolonged use. This article explores the cognitive effects of opioid pain medications and the importance of maintaining a delicate balance between pain management and cognitive well-being.

- *The Cognitive Impact:* Opioid pain medications, such as morphine, oxycodone, and hydrocodone, are known to bind to opioid receptors in the body, effectively reducing the perception of pain. However, they also have the potential to impair cognitive function. At higher doses, opioids can lead to cognitive impairment, causing individuals to experience difficulties with memory, attention, and overall cognitive performance.

- *Memory Problems:* One of the most noticeable cognitive effects of opioid use is memory problems. Individuals on opioid medications may find it challenging to retain and recall information. This can manifest as forgetfulness, the inability to remember recent events, or difficulty learning new things. For those who rely on their cognitive abilities in their daily lives, such as professionals or students, these memory problems can be particularly troublesome.

- **Reduced Cognitive Performance:** Beyond memory issues, prolonged use of opioids can result in reduced cognitive performance across the board. This includes difficulties in problem-solving, decision-making, and processing information effectively. It's crucial to recognize that while these medications can provide pain relief, they may also compromise one's ability to function at their best cognitively.

- **Balancing Act:** The key challenge in using opioid pain medications lies in balancing effective pain management and preserving cognitive function. Healthcare providers must carefully consider the dosage and duration of opioid treatment, tailoring it to the patient's specific needs. In some cases, alternative pain management strategies, such as physical therapy, non-opioid medications, or cognitive-behavioral therapy, may be explored to mitigate the cognitive risks associated with opioids.

Opioid pain medications remain valuable tools in managing pain, but their potential cognitive effects should not be underestimated. Memory problems and reduced cognitive performance can arise, especially with higher doses and prolonged use. To ensure the well-being of patients, it is essential to approach opioid use with caution, monitor cognitive function, and explore alternative pain management strategies when appropriate. The delicate balance between pain relief and brain health should always be a top priority in healthcare decisions involving opioid medications.

Medication Interactions

In some instances, interactions between multiple medications can result in cognitive side effects that may not be present when these drugs are taken individually. This underscores the importance of vigilance when it comes to polypharmacy, the practice of taking multiple medications concurrently. Healthcare providers must consider potential interactions and closely monitor cognitive function when prescribing multiple medications to a patient.

Understanding how medications impact cognitive function is essential to making informed healthcare decisions. The effects of medications on memory and cognitive abilities can vary widely, and they are not always straightforward. Suppose you are concerned about how your medications affect your memory or cognitive functions. In that case, an open and honest discussion with a healthcare professional is Important. This dialogue can lead to adjustments in your treatment plan, helping to optimize your physical and cognitive health.

Awareness of your medications' potential cognitive side effects is a proactive step toward maintaining overall health. It is imperative for individuals to discuss any concerns they may have with their healthcare providers. Medication management, dose adjustments, or even exploring alternative treatments may be considered to mitigate cognitive issues. This is especially important for those with pre-existing memory or cognitive concerns, as medication choices can significantly impact their cognitive well-being.

Monitoring cognitive function while taking medications, particularly for those with a history of memory or cognitive problems, is an ongoing process. Regular check-ins with healthcare professionals can help track any changes in cognitive function and make necessary adjustments to medication regimens.

In the journey of managing our health and well-being, knowledge and informed medication decisions play a pivotal role. By engaging in open and collaborative discussions with healthcare providers, we can make choices that address our medical needs while preserving our cognitive vitality. It's a partnership that ensures our overall well-being remains a top priority in our healthcare journey.

Reflections on Medications and Memory Interactions

The intersection of medication and memory is a multifaceted and often intricate landscape that presents both challenges and opportunities for enhancing cognitive well-being. It is truly remarkable how medications can exert both positive and negative influences on our memory and cognitive function. In today's world, where the management of multiple health conditions has become increasingly prevalent, concerns related to polypharmacy, or the concurrent use of various medications, have emerged. However, despite these concerns, there is hope that we can collectively address the risks associated with medication interactions by fostering a sense of partnership with healthcare providers and maintaining open lines of communication.

This collaborative approach holds tremendous promise in our quest to strike the right balance between effectively managing medical conditions and preserving cognitive vitality. It is widely recognized that knowledge is power, and this holds true in the realm of medications as well. Empowerment comes from actively seeking information about the drugs we are prescribed and gaining a comprehensive understanding of their potential effects on memory and cognitive function. Armed with this knowledge, we are better equipped to make informed decisions about our health, leading to a greater sense of hope and confidence in our healthcare journey.

Moreover, the invaluable collaboration between patients and healthcare providers serves as a beacon of hope in navigating the intricate relationship between medication and memory. By engaging in transparent and open communication, we can collectively make choices that not only align with our medical needs but also safeguard our cognitive vitality. This partnership allows for a holistic approach to healthcare, where the preservation of cognitive function is given due consideration alongside the management of physical ailments. The sense of hope that arises from this collaborative endeavor fuels our determination to find the optimal balance between medication management and cognitive well-being.

With hope, knowledge, and collaboration serving as guiding lights, we can envision a future where we proactively optimize both our physical and cognitive health. By staying informed, actively participating in our healthcare decisions, and fostering strong partnerships with healthcare providers, we pave the way for a brighter tomorrow—a future in which we can navigate the complex terrain of medication and memory with confidence and enjoy enhanced cognitive well-being throughout our lives.

CHAPTER 11

The Effect of Alcohol on Memory

While a drink might loosen you up, it can rob you of precious memories. Those blackouts? They're not just party anecdotes but red flags that your brain is struggling. Every forgotten night is a signal that your ability to remember, to hold onto the moments that make you, could be at risk. Choose wisely when you raise a glass—your memories are on the line.

You are not just risking a hangover when you pour that extra glass of wine or beer. You're engaging in an activity that has far-reaching consequences for your brain's health and functioning. Excessive drinking isn't merely a social faux pas; it's a gamble on your cognitive future. Memory impairments and cognitive decline are the invisible toll gates on the road of alcohol abuse.

The term Alcohol-related dementia (ARD) isn't just a scary catchphrase; it's a medical reality that demonstrates how alcohol can cause irreversible damage to your brain's architecture. Unlike other forms of dementia that may arise from genetic factors or unknown causes, ARD is directly linked to alcohol consumption.

Alcoholism acts like a time machine, but not the fun kind. It speeds up how quickly your brain ages, leading to premature cognitive decline. This accelerated aging opens the door for conditions like Wernicke-Korsakoff Syndrome, a debilitating memory disorder caused by a lack of vitamin B1, which is often deficient in people who consume alcohol excessively.

Don't be fooled; alcohol doesn't just damage the liver or heart. It also wreaks its unique havoc on the brain, a condition coined as Alcohol-Related Brain Damage (ARBD). Over time, heavy drinking can even cause your brain to shrink physically. Imagine your brain losing volume, like a balloon slowly deflating, affecting all its regions and diminishing your cognitive abilities.

But here's the sobering part—no pun intended. Even if you turn a new leaf and recover from alcohol addiction, the shadow of its impact lingers. Your risk of developing dementia remains elevated compared to those who drink moderately or abstain entirely.

So, what's the best way forward? Moderation is your friend, and complete abstinence is even better if you want to do your brain a favor. Reducing or quitting alcohol consumption can be the turning point in safeguarding your cognitive health. This change pays dividends in clarity, memory, and long-term well-being. The effects of alcohol on memory can vary depending on the amount consumed and individual factors. Here are some primary effects:

Interference with Neurotransmitters

When you consume alcohol, it doesn't just have a sedative effect; it actively interferes with the delicate balance of neurotransmitters in your brain. Neurotransmitters like glutamate and gamma-aminobutyric acid (GABA) are particularly affected. These chemical messengers are essential for the normal functioning of the nervous system and play a critical role in processes like mood regulation, motor control, and memory formation and retrieval, most notably for this discussion.

Typically, glutamate is an excitatory neurotransmitter that boosts signal transmission between neurons. Alcohol, however, suppresses the release of glutamate, leading to a general slowdown in brain activity. Conversely, GABA is an inhibitory neurotransmitter that helps to calm neural activity. Alcohol amplifies the inhibitory effects of GABA, further contributing to slowed brain functions.

So, what happens when these neurotransmitters are thrown off balance? One of the most immediate effects is impairment in memory formation. The hippocampus, a key brain area in making new memories, becomes less effective due to these neurochemical changes. This can result in short-term memory lapses, like forgetting names or losing track of time, and, in severe cases, blackouts.

In the long term, this neurotransmitter disruption can contribute to lasting memory issues and cognitive decline. The brain's plasticity, its ability to adapt and form new connections, can also be compromised. Over time, these changes can lead to noticeable deficits in cognitive abilities, not just in memory but in other functions like reasoning, planning, and problem-solving.

Therefore, understanding how alcohol interferes with neurotransmitters sheds light on the depth and complexity of its impact on the brain. This knowledge emphasizes the importance of moderation in alcohol consumption to protect both memory and overall cognitive health.

Impaired Memory Formation

When alcohol is consumed, it can have a significant impact on the brain's ability to form new memories. The intricate processes involved in memory formation are disrupted by the effects of alcohol, particularly affecting the encoding and storage of new information. To better understand this phenomenon, it can be helpful to envision the brain as a complex computer system. Under normal circumstances, the brain efficiently saves new files or memories, but when alcohol is introduced, it can lead to corruption or incompleteness in these files. It's important to note that this disruption is not limited to short-term effects; if heavy drinking persists over time, it can result in lasting issues.

The implications of impaired memory formation extend beyond simply forgetting parts of an evening or experiencing temporary lapses in memory. Instead, excessive alcohol consumption can lead to long-term cognitive difficulties. In essence, when individuals engage in heavy drinking, they not only alter their present state but also take risks with their brain's future capabilities.

Alcohol-induced memory impairment occurs through various mechanisms. Firstly, alcohol affects the communication between neurons in the brain, interfering with the efficient transmission of signals necessary for memory formation. Additionally, alcohol can disrupt the functioning of the hippocampus, a brain region crucial for forming new memories. This interference can result in fragmented or incomplete memories, making it challenging to recall events accurately.

Furthermore, chronic alcohol abuse can lead to structural changes in the brain, including shrinkage of the hippocampus and other regions involved in memory processes. Over time, these alterations can contribute to persistent cognitive difficulties, such as problems with attention, learning, and overall cognitive functioning.

It's important to recognize that the impact of alcohol on memory and cognitive function can vary depending on factors such as the amount and frequency of alcohol consumption, individual susceptibility, and overall health. However, it is generally understood that excessive and prolonged alcohol use poses risks to memory and cognitive abilities.

Understanding the potential consequences of alcohol-related memory impairment is crucial for making informed decisions about alcohol consumption. By recognizing the potential long-term implications, individuals can weigh the immediate pleasures of drinking against the possible risks to their brain health. Taking steps to moderate alcohol intake and seeking support if struggling with alcohol abuse can help mitigate the adverse effects on memory and cognition, promoting better overall brain function and preserving cognitive capabilities for the future.

Fragmented Memory Recall

A full blackout isn't the only way alcohol can mess with your memory; it can also cause fragmented memory recall, a condition where your recollection of events becomes disconnected, hazy, or even distorted, unlike a blackout where there's a complete void, fragmented memory recall leaves you with bits and pieces of the experience but not the whole picture. You may remember certain moments with clarity, like snapshots, but find it challenging to connect these fragments into a coherent story.

For example, you might recall the beginning of a night out and a few scattered events but not the order in which they happened or the context surrounding them. This can be confusing and troubling, as you're left questioning the accuracy of your memories. The reason for this phenomenon lies in how alcohol interferes with the brain's memory processes. Memory formation is a complex sequence involving encoding, storage, and retrieval. Alcohol specifically disrupts the encoding phase, making it difficult for the brain to form well-structured memories in the first place.

Additionally, the hippocampus, a region of the brain critical for memory formation, is susceptible to the effects of alcohol. When you drink, you're effectively handicapping this essential part of your brain. The implications of fragmented memory recall can be significant. For one, it compromises your ability to fully understand and remember situations, potentially affecting your decisions and behavior. It also poses questions about the reliability of your memories, which can be unsettling on a personal level. In a broader sense, experiencing fragmented memories should serve as another warning sign that alcohol affects your cognitive health and that moderation should be seriously considered.

Difficulty Retrieving Information

Consuming alcohol doesn't just affect your ability to form new memories; it can also make it challenging to access existing ones. This is known as retrieval impairment, and it can be particularly noticeable when you're trying to recall information or events that took place while you were drinking or shortly after that. For example, you might struggle to remember the name of someone you met at a party where you were drinking.

Or perhaps you read an important email while having a few drinks and later find that you can't remember its contents or even the gist of the conversation. This isn't just about the events happening while intoxicated; it's about the diminished capability of your brain to pull up information that is already stored in your memory banks. Why does this happen?

The brain's hippocampus is an indispensable player in memory formation and retrieval. Alcohol affects neurotransmitters within the hippocampus, disrupting its ability to access memories effectively. This can be both frustrating and problematic, as it impacts your ability to perform tasks that require memory recall, whether remembering a commitment you made or retrieving learned information for a work project. The issue of retrieval impairment adds another layer to the complexities of how alcohol affects cognitive health. It serves as a reminder of the immediate impairments that can occur. Excessive alcohol consumption highlights broader risks to mental functioning. This indicates that moderating alcohol consumption benefits and preserves cognitive health.

Blackouts

Blackouts from alcohol consumption go beyond simple lapses in memory. They create alarming voids in your life's timeline that you can't later fill in despite being fully active and functional at the time. Your brain falters in a vital role during these episodes: it fails to solidify these ongoing experiences into lasting memories, a process known as memory consolidation. This isn't a minor issue. It implies that you may be making impactful decisions or engaging in risky behavior without recollection.

Imagine you attend a party, and after having multiple drinks, you wake up the next day with no memory of how you got home. Friends fill you in, saying you danced, made a toast, and even engaged in a meaningful conversation. Still, you draw a blank. This is a blackout. While you were participating in activities and socializing, your brain couldn't lock in any new memories because alcohol disrupted the process of memory consolidation.

This is particularly problematic because you don't need to be a frequent heavy drinker to experience a blackout. Factors like your genetic predisposition, how tired you are, and whether you've eaten can all contribute, putting even those who drink moderately at risk. A blackout is far more than an uncomfortable gap in memory; it's a bright red flag waving at you, signaling that you may be compromising your cognitive health. It's an indispensable wake-up call, urging you to evaluate your drinking habits closely. The stakes are high; it's not just about one forgotten night but rather a signal that your brain's health could be in jeopardy.

Alcohol-Related Brain Damage (ARBD)

In social circles, alcohol often seems like the life of the party, gracing our celebrations and casual get-togethers. But beyond the well-known physical consequences of heavy drinking, such as liver issues or weight gain, lurks the lesser-known but critical impact of Alcohol-Related Brain Damage (ARBD). ARBD isn't a single condition but a range of cognitive and neurological impairments that stem from chronic, excessive alcohol consumption. These aren't momentary lapses of memory or poor judgment that you can laugh off the next day; they're lasting and often irreversible changes in your brain's functions.

The most striking feature of ARBD is its detrimental effect on memory and cognitive abilities. This impact isn't trivial; it extends to persistent forgetfulness, impaired decision-making, and emotional instability. For example, you may find yourself increasingly unable to remember new information or struggle with tasks that require planning and organization. These cognitive problems don't occur in a vacuum. They are rooted in how alcohol interferes with your brain's neurotransmitters—chemical messengers like dopamine, glutamate, and gamma-aminobutyric acid (GABA). Disruption in these neurotransmitters affects your mood and leads to more severe cognitive impairments linked with ARBD.

Diagnosing ARBD can be complex, mainly because its symptoms often mirror other cognitive disorders. You may experience anything from short-term memory gaps and difficulty concentrating to sudden, inexplicable mood swings. While some of these cognitive functions can be partially reclaimed through abstinence and supportive therapies, prevention remains the best defense. Prompt medical evaluation and intervention are indispensable if you suspect you or someone you know may be dealing with ARBD. Treatment options can include cognitive rehabilitation and medications designed to manage symptoms. Still, the most effective way to combat ARBD is by quitting alcohol.

Alcohol-related brain Damage is a serious and under-recognized consequence of heavy drinking that poses a long-term risk to your cognitive health and overall quality of life. If you believe that 'just one more drink' couldn't hurt, think again. Every drink has a lasting impact on your brain and its precious memories. So, the next time you're tempted to uncork that bottle, consider what's truly at stake: a future where your mind remains as clear and vibrant as your best days.

Wernicke-Korsakoff Syndrome

This syndrome is a debilitating neurological condition often linked to chronic alcohol abuse. However, it can also arise from other causes of severe thiamine (vitamin B1) deficiency, such as malnutrition or certain medical conditions. It comprises two interconnected disorders: Wernicke's encephalopathy and Korsakoff's psychosis.

Wernicke's encephalopathy is typically the first phase to manifest and serves as a red flag. It presents acutely with symptoms like confusion, unsteady gait, and abnormal eye movements, including nystagmus, where the eyes move uncontrollably. This stage can cause severe disorientation and impair the individual's ability to perform daily activities. Immediate medical intervention, often involving high-dose thiamine injections, can reverse these symptoms if caught early enough. However, promptly addressing it can lead to irreversible damage and may even be fatal.

Following Wernicke's encephalopathy, or sometimes occurring simultaneously, is Korsakoff's psychosis. This is a chronic condition characterized by severe memory impairments. The affected individual might find it incredibly difficult to form new memories, known as anterograde amnesia, or retrieve old ones, known as retrograde amnesia. Interestingly, a person with Korsakoff's psychosis may engage in "confabulation," where they fill in memory gaps with fabricated stories, often without realizing that they are doing so.

The long-term effects of Wernicke-Korsakoff Syndrome can be profoundly life-altering. Beyond memory issues, other cognitive functions like reasoning, problem-solving, and planning can deteriorate. Social relationships often suffer, as do vocational capabilities, making regular employment challenging. The syndrome often necessitates long-term care and supervision, which can emotionally and financially drain families.

DAVID L. PRIEDE, PHD

Prevention remains the most effective strategy for Wernicke-Korsakoff Syndrome. Abstaining from excessive alcohol consumption and maintaining a balanced diet rich in essential nutrients, like vitamin B1, can significantly lower the risk. Even in chronic alcohol users, supplementing with thiamine can provide a layer of protection against the development of this debilitating syndrome.

Wernicke-Korsakoff Syndrome is a devastating, often irreversible neurological condition primarily brought on by chronic alcohol abuse and thiamine deficiency. Its impacts extend beyond memory impairment, affecting multiple facets of cognition and dramatically diminishing the quality of life.

Long-Term Effects of Alcohol Consumption

The impact of alcohol on your brain isn't limited to just the immediate short-term effects like blackouts or fragmented memories; it can also have lingering, long-term consequences. Persistent, heavy drinking can permanently alter your brain structure, damaging memory, and various cognitive functions.

These structural brain changes can manifest in several ways. For example, neuroimaging studies have shown that chronic alcohol abuse can reduce the size of the hippocampus, a critical brain region for memory formation and retrieval. Smaller hippocampal volume is associated with impaired memory and cognitive function. Furthermore, chronic drinking can affect the integrity of the brain's white matter, which is essential for efficient neural communication. Deterioration of white matter can lead to issues with attention, problem-solving, and decision-making.

Conditions like Alcohol-Related Brain Damage (ARBD) and Wernicke-Korsakoff Syndrome, a severe memory disorder caused by a lack of vitamin B1, can also develop from long-term alcohol abuse. These conditions are often irreversible and can drastically reduce quality of life, affecting not just the individual but their families and communities.

Even after periods of abstinence or sobriety, the risks can persist. People with a history of alcohol abuse are at a heightened risk for developing conditions like dementia later in life. This shows that the brain may not fully recover from the harmful effects of excessive alcohol consumption, underscoring the importance of moderation or abstinence as a preventive measure to maintain cognitive health.

Understanding these long-term implications is key for anyone considering their drinking habits, as it's not just about the risk of a hangover or a forgotten night. It's about the lasting impact on your brain and, by extension, your life.

Reflections on The Effect of Alcohol on Memory

If safeguarding your memory and overall brainpower matters to you, then it's time to get honest about your relationship with alcohol. Think of alcohol as the friend who talks you into questionable decisions, like texting your ex at midnight or buying that neon-green jumpsuit you'll never wear. Just like that friend, alcohol can mess with your cognitive judgment, particularly when it comes to memory.

So, what can you do? You have choices: consider scaling back drinking or avoiding alcohol altogether, especially if you find you're prone to memory issues after a night of cocktails or beers. It's not just about saving face by remembering names at parties or where you left your keys. It's about preserving the health of your brain in the long term—because, let's face it, you're going to need it!

And if you're already noticing that your memory is taking a hit due to excessive drinking, don't despair or try to navigate the rocky terrain alone. There's help available, whether it's from medical professionals, addiction specialists, or support groups. Reaching out for expert advice isn't a sign of defeat; it's an empowered step towards reclaiming your cognitive health and, by extension, your life. So, if you or someone you love is grappling with alcohol misuse, don't just sit there and let your brain suffer. Act now; your future self will thank you.

CHAPTER 12

The Connection Between Weight and Memory

Your weight goes beyond physical health, as it may affect cognitive function with links to diminished cerebral blood flow and potential risks to reasoning and memory. Fortunately, weight loss interventions, encompassing dietary adjustments and regular exercise, play a pivotal role in shaping one's physique and mitigating and enhancing cognitive faculties for a more resilient and focused future.

O besity is not just an epidemic of the body; it's also becoming a crisis for the mind. As fast-food joints and processed snacks dominate our diets, the problem extends beyond aesthetics and physical well-being. Increasingly, research demonstrates that obesity has severe implications for brain health, specifically cognitive functioning. Many may not realize that obesity hampers the efficiency of blood flow throughout the body, leading to decreased cerebral blood flow (CBF). Good blood flow to the brain is not merely a physiological luxury; it's necessary for cognitive functions like reasoning, memory retention, and attention span.

The relationship between obesity and decreased CBF should ring alarm bells. This reduced blood flow can inhibit the brain's ability to function optimally, affecting decision-making processes and memory recall.

What makes this especially worrying is the long-term impact. Studies have shown that carrying excess weight during your middle years significantly elevates your risk of developing debilitating cognitive conditions like dementia in later life. Therefore, it becomes paramount to see obesity not just as a condition affecting physical well-being but as a dire threat to mental acuity and cognitive longevity.

Weight loss interventions aren't just about looking good or reducing the strain on your heart; they're about reclaiming your mental faculties. Encouragingly, research has shown that cognitive functions can improve with weight loss in individuals who are overweight or obese. These interventions can range from dietary changes to incorporating regular exercise into one's routine, all aimed at reversing the cognitive decline associated with obesity. Given the clear and alarming linkage between excess weight and cognitive degeneration, there has never been a more compelling reason to maintain a healthy weight. Your brain, that incredible organ that defines who you are, relies on you to make the right choices today for a sharper, more focused tomorrow.

The effects of obesity on memory are a growing concern in the modern world. Obesity can have several adverse effects on memory and cognitive function, including:

- *Reduced Cerebral Blood Flow:* Obesity is associated with decreased cerebral blood flow (CBF), affecting the brain's ability to function optimally. Adequate CBF is essential for memory, attention, and overall cognitive performance.
- *Inflammation:* Obesity is often accompanied by chronic low-grade inflammation. Inflammatory processes in the body can extend to the brain, potentially leading to cognitive impairments, including memory problems.
- *Insulin Resistance:* Obesity is a common risk factor for insulin resistance and type 2 diabetes. Insulin plays a role in brain function, and insulin resistance may negatively impact memory and cognitive abilities.
- *Hormonal Changes:* Obesity can lead to hormonal imbalances, including alterations in hormones like leptin and adiponectin, which regulate appetite and metabolism. These hormonal changes may influence brain function and memory.
- *Structural Brain Changes:* Studies have shown that obesity can lead to structural changes in the brain, including alterations in the hippocampus, a region Important for memory formation. These changes may contribute to memory deficits.
- *Sleep Disturbances:* Obesity is a risk factor for sleep apnea and other sleep disorders. Poor sleep quality or sleep disturbances can impair memory consolidation and cognitive function.
- *Vascular Factors:* Obesity is associated with an increased risk of cardiovascular diseases, including hypertension and atherosclerosis. Vascular conditions can

impair blood flow to the brain, potentially affecting memory.

- **Psychosocial Factors:** The psychosocial consequences of obesity, such as depression, low self-esteem, and social isolation, can contribute to cognitive and memory problems.
- **Alzheimer's Disease Risk:** Some studies suggest that obesity in midlife is associated with a higher risk of developing Alzheimer's disease later in life. Alzheimer's is characterized by significant memory decline.
- **Executive Function Impairment:** Executive function refers to a set of cognitive processes responsible for planning, decision-making, problem-solving, and self-control. Obesity has been associated with impairments in executive function, which can impact various aspects of daily life and cognitive abilities.
- **Gut Microbiota Imbalances:** Emerging research suggests that the gut microbiota, the community of microorganisms residing in the digestive tract, may play a role in the relationship between obesity and cognitive function. Imbalances in the gut microbiota, often observed in obesity, have been linked to cognitive impairments and memory problems.
- **Effects on Neurotransmitters:** Obesity can disrupt the balance of neurotransmitters in the brain, such as dopamine and serotonin, which are involved in mood regulation and cognitive processes. These disruptions may contribute to memory impairments and cognitive decline.
- **Impact on Brain Aging:** Obesity has been associated with accelerated brain aging, characterized by a decline in cognitive function and an increased risk of neurodegenerative diseases. Exploring the mechanisms through which obesity accelerates brain aging can provide valuable insights into the link between obesity and cognitive decline.

Obesity, characterized by excessive body weight and a high body mass index (BMI), has been linked to various health concerns, including an increased risk of cardiovascular disease, diabetes, and certain cancers. In recent years, research has also shed light on the impact of obesity on cognitive function, including memory.

The relationship between obesity and memory is intricate and influenced by multiple factors. One contributing factor is the chronic low-grade inflammation often associated with obesity. This inflammation can affect the structure and function of the brain, including regions involved in memory processes. Additionally, obesity is associated with insulin resistance and metabolic dysfunction, which can impair brain health and cognitive function, including memory.

However, it's important to emphasize that individual responses to obesity and its impact on memory can vary. Some individuals with obesity may not experience significant memory impairments, while others may be more susceptible. Genetic factors, lifestyle choices, and overall health status can all influence the extent to which obesity affects memory.

Fortunately, adopting a healthier lifestyle can help mitigate some of the adverse effects of obesity on memory and cognitive function. Regular physical activity has been shown to have positive effects on brain health, including improved memory and cognitive performance. Engaging in activities that elevate heart rate and increase blood flow to the brain, such as aerobic exercises, can be particularly beneficial.

A balanced diet is also crucial for both weight management and optimal brain function. Nutrient-rich foods, including fruits, vegetables, whole grains, and lean proteins, provide essential vitamins, minerals, and antioxidants that support brain health. In contrast, a diet high in saturated fats, added sugars, and processed foods may contribute to cognitive decline and memory impairments.

Weight management plays a vital role in mitigating the effects of obesity on memory. Achieving and maintaining a healthy weight through a combination of regular physical activity and a balanced diet can help reduce inflammation, improve insulin sensitivity, and enhance overall brain function.

Moreover, addressing other risk factors associated with obesity, such as hypertension and sleep apnea, can also positively impact memory and cognitive health. Managing these comorbidities through appropriate medical interventions and lifestyle modifications can contribute to better brain function.

While the relationship between obesity and memory is complex, adopting a healthier lifestyle that includes regular physical activity, a balanced diet, and weight management can help mitigate some of the adverse effects.

By maintaining a healthy weight, addressing related risk factors, and promoting overall brain health, individuals can improve memory preservation and enhance cognitive function. It's essential

106

to consult with healthcare professionals for personalized guidance and support in managing obesity and its potential impact on memory.

Obesity, Genetic Factors, and Cultural Influences

Obesity is a multifaceted issue influenced by a combination of genetic factors and cultural influences. Genetic factors play a significant role in determining an individual's susceptibility to obesity. Research has identified specific genes associated with obesity, including those involved in regulating appetite, metabolism, and fat storage. Individuals with certain genetic variations may have a higher predisposition to gaining weight or experiencing difficulties in weight management. However, it's important to note that genetics alone do not dictate one's weight or risk of obesity. Cultural influences and environmental factors also play a crucial role. Cultural norms, traditions, and societal attitudes toward food and physical activity can greatly impact an individual's eating habits, lifestyle choices, and overall health.

Genetic Foundations

Genetic predispositions determine how individuals interact with their environment, particularly concerning weight-related challenges such as obesity. Genetic research has uncovered specific genetic markers and familial patterns that contribute significantly to an individual's predisposition for obesity.

These genetic markers are variations in the DNA sequence that can influence factors like metabolism, appetite regulation, and fat storage. For instance, certain gene variants may make an individual more prone to storing excess calories as fat, while others may affect how efficiently the body burns calories. Familial patterns highlight the hereditary aspect of obesity, demonstrating that individuals with a family history of obesity are more likely to share similar genetic factors contributing to their susceptibility.

Understanding these genetic predispositions provides valuable insights into the variability observed in individuals' responses to external factors such as diet and physical activity. While genetics alone does not determine an individual's destiny in terms of weight, it sets the stage for how their body might respond to environmental influences. This knowledge is essential for tailoring personalized approaches to weight management, considering the unique genetic factors that may influence an individual's propensity to develop obesity.

Cultural Perspectives

Exploring cultural influences unveils a rich tapestry of factors that intricately shape individuals' lifestyle choices, dietary habits, and physical activity levels. Cultural norms and traditions, deeply embedded in the fabric of societies, play a pivotal role in determining how people relate to food and exercise. This investigation extends beyond individual behaviors, considering the broader societal structures influencing health-related decisions.

Cultural perceptions of body image wield significant influence, dictating societal ideals and beauty standards. These perceptions often contribute to developing specific attitudes towards food, exercise, and body weight. Societal expectations, influenced by cultural norms, can create positive and negative pressures, impacting individuals' choices regarding their health and well-being. The interplay of cultural factors also extends to economic considerations, as access to nutritious food, recreational facilities, and healthcare resources may vary across different communities.

By understanding how cultural perceptions, societal expectations, and economic factors intersect, we gain insights into the diverse challenges communities worldwide face in addressing and mitigating the impact of obesity. This exploration paves the way for comprehensive strategies that consider the cultural context in promoting healthier lifestyles and combating the multifaceted nature of the obesity epidemic.

Navigating Solutions

A nuanced comprehension of genetic and cultural factors is imperative for designing effective public health interventions targeting the obesity epidemic. By discerning the intricate interplay between genetic predispositions and cultural influences, interventions can be tailored to specific populations, acknowledging their unique challenges and susceptibilities. Understanding the genetic markers associated with obesity allows for targeted prevention strategies, while cultural insights enable the development of interventions that resonate with diverse communities.

Education emerges as a powerful tool in reshaping food and exercising cultural norms. By fostering awareness and promoting informed choices, educational initiatives can influence behavioral patterns and contribute to healthier lifestyles. Integrating culturally sensitive educational programs ensures that interventions align with diverse beliefs and practices, fostering greater community acceptance and engagement. By adopting a comprehensive perspective, we strive to promote sustainable health outcomes and foster a collective effort towards combating obesity on both genetic and cultural fronts.

Reflections on The Connection Between Weight and Memory

Exploring the correlation between weight and memory delves into understanding how carrying extra weight may influence our ability to remember effectively. It transcends merely viewing weight as a numerical value on a scale; rather, it involves recognizing it as a variable that could intricately shape the storage and retrieval processes within our brains.

In this endeavor, our aim is to comprehend the potential alterations in functioning that accompany increased body weight. This entails delving into the underlying mechanisms at play when we accumulate additional pounds. Rather than relying on convoluted terminology, our focus lies in untangling the ways in which our body shape might impact our memory capabilities.

This endeavor mirrors the process of solving a complex puzzle, where we endeavor to establish meaningful connections between our physical stature and the memories that contribute to our sense of self. Through this exploration, we gain insights into how our weight could potentially influence our memory function, akin to uncovering a hidden pathway within the vast realm of scientific inquiry.

Ultimately, this journey of exploration leads to a deeper understanding of the intricate interplay between our bodily state and cognitive processes. It serves as a pathway to unlocking new perspectives and insights into the interconnectedness between our physicality and the functioning of our memory.

CHAPTER 13

How Socializing Boosts Memory

Socializing unveils a remarkable link between human connections and memory enhancement. Beyond casual conversations, social interactions become a potent elixir for memory challenges, creating vibrant neural connections that fortify memory recall. This dynamic dance between socializing and memory isn't just a remedy; it's a canvas where each interaction contributes to cognitive resilience.

Engaging in social activities and maintaining social connections benefits memory and cognition. However, how we socialize has undergone significant changes with the advent of technology and the prevalence of digital interactions. This technological shift has brought about positive and negative consequences for our cognitive processes. On the positive side, the digital age has granted us unprecedented access to a vast reservoir of information and stimuli. However, it has also contributed to the widespread phenomenon of shortened attention spans among many individuals constantly immersed in digital interactions.

Nevertheless, primarily through language and communication, socializing plays a pivotal role in shaping our cognitive health. Language use facilitates communication, fosters cognitive development, and even contributes to forming our identities. Moreover, social interaction can serve as a protective factor, slowing the onset of dementia in aging individuals. In essence, staying socially engaged is yet another activity that keeps our brains active and functioning optimally.

Benefits of Social Activity and Memory

Engaging in social activities has a profound impact on cognitive health, with recent research findings supporting and enhancing various aspects:

- *Cognitive Stimulation:* Social interactions often involve engaging in conversations, problem-solving, and sharing experiences. These activities provide cognitive stimulation that can help maintain and enhance memory function.

- **Reduced Risk of Cognitive Decline:** Socially active Individuals have a reduced risk of cognitive decline and memory problems as they age. Regular social engagement may delay the onset of conditions like dementia and Alzheimer's disease.
- **Emotional Support:** Social connections provide emotional support, reducing stress and anxiety. Chronic stress can negatively affect memory and cognitive function, so having a strong social support system can be protective.
- **Enhanced Brain Plasticity:** Social activities can promote brain plasticity, the brain's ability to adapt and reorganize itself. Engaging with others, learning from different perspectives, and participating in new experiences can improve cognitive flexibility and memory.
- **Improved Mood:** Positive social interactions often improve mood and overall well-being. A positive mood is associated with better cognitive performance, including memory.
- **Sense of Purpose:** Social engagement gives individuals a sense of purpose and belonging, which can positively influence their overall mental health and cognitive resilience.
- **Brain Health Benefits:** Studies have indicated that socializing may increase brain volume in areas associated with memory and cognitive function. This suggests a direct link between social activity and brain health.
- **Lifelong Learning:** Interacting with a diverse group of people exposes individuals to new ideas and perspectives, encouraging lifelong learning. Continuous learning has been associated with better cognitive outcomes, including memory retention.
- **Maintaining An Active Social Life:** This profoundly impacts memory and cognitive health. Social activities provide mental stimulation, emotional support, and opportunities for personal growth, all of which contribute to better memory retention and a reduced risk of memory-related conditions. For individuals concerned about memory loss or cognitive decline, staying socially engaged is a valuable strategy to promote brain health and overall well-being.

Impacts of Technology on Socialization and Cognition Across Ages, Cultures, and Socioeconomic Levels

Engaging in social activities and maintaining connections is essential for memory and cognition. Still, the impact of technology on socialization and cognition varies significantly among different age groups, cultural backgrounds, and socioeconomic statuses. Considering these diverse perspectives adds depth to our understanding of how technology influences our cognitive processes.

In the digital age, where information and stimuli are readily accessible, there is a notable difference in how various age groups adapt to and are affected by constant digital interactions. Younger generations, often referred to as digital natives, may find it easier to navigate and benefit from the positive aspects of technology, such as vast information access.

On the other hand, older individuals may face challenges in adjusting to the rapid changes, potentially experiencing drawbacks such as shortened attention spans.

Cultural backgrounds also play a critical role in shaping the impact of technology on socialization and cognition. Different cultures may have varying attitudes toward digital interactions, affecting how individuals within those cultures engage socially. Some cultures may embrace technology for communication and information-sharing, while others may prioritize traditional forms of socialization.

Socioeconomic status further influences the dynamics of technology use. Individuals with higher socioeconomic statuses might have greater access to advanced digital technologies and resources, potentially experiencing different cognitive effects compared to those with limited access. Socioeconomic disparities can also influence the quality and quantity of social interactions facilitated by technology.

Considering these diverse perspectives is vital in understanding how technology shapes cognitive health through social activities. By recognizing the variations among age groups, cultural backgrounds, and socioeconomic statuses, we can better tailor discussions and interventions to address the specific needs and challenges faced by different segments of the population. Ultimately, an inclusive approach ensures that the benefits and drawbacks of technology on memory and cognition are understood in a holistic and context-sensitive manner.

Potential Challenges and Limitations

While social activity offers numerous benefits, it is essential to acknowledge potential challenges and limitations to provide a comprehensive perspective:

- **Cognitive Overload:** Extensive exposure to social interactions, especially in the digital realm, may lead to cognitive overload. Continuous notifications and information influx can overwhelm individuals, affecting their cognitive processes negatively.
- **Impaired Attention:** Technology, including social media, can contribute to attention-related issues. Notifications and constant connectivity may result in heightened attention-deficit symptoms, impacting cognitive focus and performance.
- **Reduced Face-to-Face Interaction:** Over-reliance on digital communication might diminish face-to-face social interactions. This shift can have implications for emotional intelligence and the nuanced understanding derived from in-person communication.
- **Social Isolation:** Paradoxically, excessive use of technology may lead to social isolation. Individuals may prioritize online interactions over real-world connections, impacting the richness of social engagement and emotional support.

Balancing the discussion by acknowledging these challenges ensures a nuanced understanding of the complex relationship between social activity and cognitive processes.

How to Improve Attention Span in The Digital Age

To improve attention span in the digital age, individuals can consider the following strategies:

- **Minimize Distractions:** Limiting exposure to distractions, such as turning off non-essential notifications and creating a conducive work environment, can help individuals maintain focus and attention
- **Interactive Learning:** Incorporating interactive learning methods, such as multimedia, simulations, and

gamification, can capture attention through visual and kinesthetic learning

- *Microlearning:* Utilizing microlearning techniques, such as short videos, infographics, and quizzes, can help individuals absorb information in small, manageable chunks, making learning more digestible and engaging
- *Collaborative Learning:* Engaging in more collaborative and social learning through discussions, group projects, and peer-to-peer activities can promote active engagement and encourage learning from one another
- *Real-World Relevance:* Relating concepts to real-world examples and applications that demonstrate relevance to individuals' lives can increase motivation and interest, thus sustaining attention
- *Educational Technology:* Leveraging educational technology for personalized and self-paced learning can help tailor the learning journey to each individual's unique pace and preferences, thus maintaining engagement
- *Active Listening:* Practicing active listening can help individuals improve their ability to focus without letting unnecessary distractions interrupt their work or conversations
- *Exercise:* Engaging in physical exercise has been shown to improve attention span and overall cognitive function
- *Meditation:* Incorporating meditation into daily routines can help individuals enhance their ability to maintain focus and reduce the impact of external distractions on attention span
- *Limit Multitasking:* Avoiding multitasking and focusing on one task at a time can help individuals maintain sustained attention during activities.

By implementing these strategies, individuals can work towards improving their attention span in the digital age and enhancing their overall cognitive performance.

Reflections on How Socializing Boosts Memory

Socializing serves as a potent catalyst for both mental well-being and cognitive enhancement. It's not merely about enjoying good company; it's also a significant memory booster. Engaging in conversations, sharing laughs, and participating in social activities do more than just pass the time pleasantly—they actively stimulate brain regions responsible for memory, such as the hippocampus.

The social brain hypothesis posits that our brains have evolved to excel in social environments, and this natural inclination toward socialization enhances memory formation.

When we share memorable moments with friends or family, we're creating a rich tapestry of interconnected memories. Whether it's a birthday celebration, a holiday gathering, or a casual outing, these shared experiences are not just fleeting moments but contribute to the fabric of our long-term memory. Socializing also involves learning from others, which can enhance cognitive flexibility and adaptability, allowing us to better navigate various situations and challenges.

The benefits of social interaction are not confined to in-person encounters. Virtual socialization through technology also has a significant role to play. Meaningful connections, whether physical or digital, can ignite cognitive processes that reinforce and fortify our memory. In the digital age, even online interactions can provide the cognitive engagement necessary to stimulate the brain.

Therefore, the next time you engage in social activities, remember that you're doing more than just creating enjoyable experiences. You're actively participating in a process that boosts your memory prowess. Socializing helps reduce stress and depression, and it also serves as a powerful tool for cognitive enhancement, contributing to a healthier, more resilient mind.

CHAPTER 14

The Role of Vision, Hearing, Taste, Smell, and Touch in Memory

As we age, our sensory abilities, including hearing, vision, taste, smell, and touch, can diminish, posing additional challenges to our cognitive journey. Hearing and vision problems can strain the brain and impact memory, while changes in taste, smell, and touch sensitivity can affect daily experiences and interactions. These alterations in sensory perception contribute to the multifaceted nature of cognitive challenges associated with aging.

The aging process affects our brains and our bodies, and these physical changes can directly impact the brain's aging. One of the most common signs of biological aging is the gradual decline in our sensory abilities, particularly regarding hearing and vision. These age-related sensory impairments can play a significant role in the deterioration of memory and cognitive function.

Untreated vision problems, for example, can also strain cognitive resources, particularly when individuals struggle to see and interpret visual information. The brain's efforts to compensate for vision impairments can divert cognitive resources from memory and tasks, further exacerbating cognitive difficulties. For instance, imagine a world traveler with untreated vision problems exploring breathtaking destinations.

Their impaired vision hinders their whole experience of vibrant landscapes and hues. As time passes, the memories of these experiences lose their vividness, devoid of the vibrant colors that undiminished sight would have provided. Untreated vision problems diminish the clarity and visual impact of cherished memories, leaving behind faded impressions of remarkable destinations.

Similarly, untreated hearing loss can lead to cognitive difficulties. When the brain must strain to process sounds due to hearing impairment, it allocates more cognitive resources to this task, leaving fewer resources available for memory and other cognitive processes. For example, untreated hearing loss affects the memories of a person attending a loved one's wedding. Their inability to fully experience the music, laughter, and speeches due to hearing impairment diminishes the vibrancy and detail of their recollection over time. The untreated hearing loss diminishes the clarity and impact of their cherished memory of the wedding.

Taste, or gustation, refers to the perception of different flavors and is closely linked to memory. Recognizing and remembering specific tastes is necessary for survival and developing preferences and aversions towards certain foods. The sense of taste can evoke powerful emotional and sensory experiences that become associated with specific memories. For example, the taste of a favorite childhood dish may bring back vivid memories of family gatherings or special occasions.

Similarly, the sense of smell, or olfaction, is strongly linked to memory and emotion. The olfactory system is unique in its direct connection to the brain's limbic system, which is involved in memory and emotion processing. The olfactory memories we form are often highly evocative and can transport us back to specific moments. For instance, catching a whiff of a familiar perfume or the aroma of freshly baked cookies can trigger vivid memories and emotions associated with those smells.

Touch, or the somatosensory system, also contributes to memory in various ways. The sensation of touch is closely tied to our experiences of texture, temperature, pressure, and pain. These tactile sensations can create lasting memories and associations. For example, the touch of a loved one, the feel of a soft fabric, or the pain of a burn all leave imprints in our memory. Additionally, tactile information can enhance memory encoding and retrieval. Studies have shown that physical touch during learning or recall can improve memory performance.

However, the key takeaway is that appropriate treatment can make a significant difference. By proactively addressing these age-related sensory changes, individuals can enhance their overall cognitive health and maintain their memory and cognitive abilities as they age.

How Sensory Functions Affect Memory

Sensory functions play a central role in memory formation and retrieval. Our senses, such as vision, hearing, taste, smell, and touch, provide us with the information we need to perceive and understand the world around us. Here's how sensory functions affect memory:

- *Visual input:* The Visual system processes visual information, including the eyes and the brain's visual cortex. Visual stimuli can be highly influential in memory formation. For example, vivid and detailed visual images or scenes are often easier to remember than abstract or less visually distinctive information. Visual cues can trigger the retrieval of associated memories, as our visual system is adept at recognizing and recalling visual patterns, faces, and objects.

- *Auditory input:* Auditory information, such as sounds and speech, is processed by the auditory system, including the ears and the auditory cortex of the brain. Auditory cues can have a powerful impact on memory formation and retrieval. For instance, hearing a particular sound or a familiar voice can evoke memories of past experiences linked to that sound. Additionally, verbal information heard through speech can be encoded and stored in memory, facilitating later retrieval.

- *Olfactory input:* The sense of smell, processed by the olfactory system, can strongly influence memory. Smells have a unique ability to evoke powerful emotional and memory associations. Specific odors can trigger vivid recollections of past events, people, or places. This phenomenon is due to the close anatomical connection between the olfactory system and the brain regions responsible for memory and emotion, such as the hippocampus and the amygdala.

- *Taste input:* The sense of taste, processed by the tongue's taste buds, is also closely linked to memory formation. The flavors and tastes of food or other substances can create strong memory associations. This is particularly evident when taste is connected to emotional experiences or significant events, such as the taste of a favorite childhood treat or a memorable meal.

- *Tactile input:* The sense of touch, including sensations of pressure, texture, and temperature, also contributes to memory formation. The tactile system, spread throughout the body, helps encode memories associated with physical sensations and experiences. The tactile cues from objects or events can be stored in memory and later retrieved, enhancing our recollection of past experiences.

Sensory Memory: Perception and Memory Formation

Sensory functions play a crucial role in memory formation and retrieval. Our senses, such as vision, hearing, taste, smell, and touch, provide us with the information we need to perceive and understand the world around us. Here's how sensory functions affect memory:

- *Encoding:* Sensory information acts as input for memory formation. When we perceive something through our senses, the sensory stimuli are encoded and processed by the brain. Different sensory modalities may be involved in encoding different aspects of a memory. For example, visual information might be necessary for remembering the appearance of an object, while auditory details might be necessary for remembering a conversation.
- *Attention:* Sensory stimuli help to direct our attention to specific details or events. Attention is a selective process that determines which sensory inputs are processed more deeply and are more likely to be remembered. For example, suppose you are paying close attention to a lecture. In that case, you are more likely to remember the information presented than if you are distracted or not actively engaged in the sensory experience.
- *Sensory cues:* Sensory cues can trigger memory retrieval. Memories are often associated with the context in which they were formed, including the sensory cues present at the time. When we encounter similar sensory cues later, they can serve as retrieval cues, prompting the recall of associated memories. For example, the smell of freshly baked cookies may trigger memories of baking with your grandmother.
- *Sensory vividness:* Memories associated with intense sensory experiences are often more vivid and easier to recall. Sensory-rich experiences tend to create more robust and detailed memory traces. For instance, emotional events that evoke strong sensory reactions, such as a traumatic incident or an exhilarating adventure, are often remembered more vividly than mundane events.

- **Sensory memory:** Sensory memory refers to the brief retention of sensory information after a stimulus is no longer present. It allows us to hold sensory impressions for a short period, typically less than a second. Although sensory memory has a limited capacity and duration, it provides a temporary buffer to transfer sensory information to other memory systems, such as short-term and long-term memory.

Overall, sensory functions provide the foundation for memory formation, influencing how information is encoded, attended to, and retrieved. By understanding the relationship between sensory experiences and memory, we can optimize learning and recall by engaging multiple senses and creating meaningful associations with the information we want to remember.

The Sensory Symphony

Memory, a captivating mosaic of our past, is intricately shaped by the convergence of our senses, where our senses intertwine, painting vivid memories with the brushstrokes of vision, sound, touch, taste, and smell. As we navigate further, we encounter the delicate balance of the fusion of senses, cognitive intricacies, and emotional resonance that form the tapestry of our memories.

Multisensory Integration

Multisensory integration is the process by which information from different sensory modalities, such as vision, hearing, and touch, is combined and integrated in the brain. This integration enhances memory formation and retrieval by creating a richer and more comprehensive representation of an experience. When multiple senses are simultaneously engaged, the brain forms stronger associations between the sensory cues and the encoded memories. For example, if you attend a concert and not only hear the music but also see the performers and feel the vibrations of the bass, the integration of these sensory inputs can create a more robust and vivid memory of the event.

Cognitive Load

Cognitive load refers to the amount of mental effort or resources required to perform a task. It has a significant impact on memory processes. When cognitive load is high, such as when trying to process complex information or juggle multiple tasks simultaneously, it can interfere with memory encoding and retrieval. The limited cognitive resources can be consumed by the task at hand, leaving fewer resources available for effective memory formation. For example, suppose you are trying to listen to a lecture while simultaneously engaging in a challenging mental calculation. In that case, the cognitive load imposed by the calculation can hinder your ability to encode and retain the lecture content in long-term memory.

Emotional Impact

Emotions play a fundamental role in memory formation and retrieval. Emotional experiences tend to be more memorable compared to neutral experiences. This phenomenon is known as the emotional enhancement effect. Emotions can enhance memory through multiple mechanisms.

For instance, emotional arousal can increase the release of neurotransmitters, such as adrenaline and noradrenaline, which can strengthen memory consolidation. Emotions also act as effective retrieval cues, facilitating the recall of memories associated with the emotional event.

Additionally, the amygdala, a brain region involved in processing emotions, interacts with memory-related brain structures, such as the hippocampus, further influencing memory formation and retrieval. Thus, events that elicit strong emotional responses are often more deeply encoded and more readily recalled.

Treatment Types and Benefits for Sensory Loss

Sensory loss can significantly impact an individual's perception, cognition, and memory, posing challenges in daily life and overall well-being. However, advancements in technology and medicine have brought forth many promising treatment options that offer hope and an improved quality of life for individuals experiencing sensory deficits.

The latest advances in technology and medicine showcase how these innovations are revolutionizing the field and providing new avenues for sensory rehabilitation and memory enhancement. From cutting-edge therapies that leverage virtual reality and neural interfaces to groundbreaking medical interventions like cochlear implants and retinal prostheses, the transformative potential of these advancements is remarkable in supporting individuals with sensory loss and improving their cognitive well-being.

For instance, advancements in assistive technologies, such as smart glasses and hearing aids with artificial intelligence capabilities, are enhancing sensory perception and cognitive function by providing real-time information processing and environmental cues. Additionally, developments in gene therapy and stem cell research hold promise for treating underlying conditions that contribute to sensory deficits, potentially restoring or improving sensory function.

With ongoing research and collaboration across disciplines, these advancements in technology and medicine are paving the way for more personalized and effective treatments, empowering individuals with sensory loss to overcome challenges and unlock their full potential. The continued progress in this field not only offers hope but also underscores the remarkable resilience of the human spirit in adapting and thriving in the face of adversity.

Hearing Loss Treatments

Hearing loss can significantly impact communication, social interactions, and overall quality of life. However, several effective treatments are available to address hearing loss and improve auditory function. The choice of treatment depends on the type and severity of hearing loss and individual preferences. Here are some common hearing loss treatments:

- *Hearing Aids:* Hearing aids are the most common and widely used treatment for hearing loss. These small electronic devices are worn in or behind the ear and amplify sound to make it more audible for the wearer. Modern hearing aids utilize advanced digital signal processing technology to provide customized amplification and improve speech intelligibility. They can be programmed to adapt to different listening environments, reduce background noise, and enhance the perception of specific frequencies. Hearing aids come in various styles and sizes to suit individual needs and preferences.

- *Cochlear Implants:* Cochlear implants are advanced medical devices designed for individuals with severe to profound hearing loss who do not benefit from hearing aids. Unlike hearing aids that amplify sound, cochlear implants bypass the damaged parts of the inner ear (cochlea) and directly stimulate the auditory nerve. The system consists of an external speech processor worn behind the ear, capturing and processing sound, and an internal implant surgically placed under the skin. The implant sends electrical signals to the auditory nerve, allowing individuals to perceive sound. Cochlear implants are particularly effective for individuals with severe sensorineural hearing loss.

- **Bone-Anchored Hearing Systems (BAHS)**: BAHS are implantable devices primarily used for individuals with conductive or mixed hearing loss or single-sided deafness. They work by transmitting sound vibrations through the skull bone to the inner ear, bypassing the outer and middle ear. BAHS consist of a small titanium implant placed in the bone behind the ear, a sound processor that attaches to the implant, and a sound-conducting abutment or an external magnet that connects the processor to the implant. BAHS can improve sound perception and speech understanding in individuals with specific types of hearing loss.

- **Middle Ear Implants:** Middle ear implants are surgically implanted devices that directly stimulate the middle ear structures to improve hearing. They are typically used for individuals who cannot use or benefit from conventional hearing aids due to certain ear conditions or anatomical factors. Middle ear implants consist of an external audio processor that captures and processes sound and an implanted component that mechanically stimulates the middle ear structures. These implants can amplify and enhance sound quality for individuals with specific types of hearing loss.

- **Assistive Listening Devices (ALDs):** ALDs are devices designed to improve hearing in specific listening situations. They work by capturing sound from a source (such as a microphone or audio system) and delivering it directly to the ear of the listener. ALDs include devices such as personal FM systems, loop systems, and infrared systems. ALDs can be beneficial when background noise or distance from the sound source makes hearing and understanding speech challenging.

It is important to consult an audiologist or hearing healthcare professional to determine the most suitable treatment option based on individual needs, hearing loss characteristics, and lifestyle considerations. They can provide a comprehensive evaluation, recommend appropriate interventions, and offer ongoing support and follow-up care to ensure optimal hearing outcomes.

Vision Loss Treatments

Vision loss can significantly impact daily functioning and quality of life. While some causes of vision loss may be irreversible, treatments and interventions are available to manage vision loss, improve remaining vision, and enhance independence. The specific treatment options depend on the underlying cause and severity of vision loss. Here are some common treatments for vision loss:

- **Corrective Lenses:** Corrective lenses, such as eyeglasses or contact lenses, are the most common and straightforward treatment for refractive errors like nearsightedness, farsightedness, and astigmatism. They can help improve visual acuity and clarity by compensating for the abnormalities in the eye's focusing power. An eye care professional can prescribe the appropriate lenses based on an individual's specific visual needs.

- **Medications:** In some cases, vision loss may be caused by underlying conditions that can be managed or stabilized with medication. For example, certain eye conditions like glaucoma, macular degeneration, or diabetic retinopathy may be treated with eye drops, oral medications, or injections to slow down disease progression or manage symptoms. It is essential to consult with an ophthalmologist or eye specialist to determine the most suitable medication options.

- **Low Vision Devices:** Low vision devices can benefit individuals with significant vision loss or conditions that cannot be fully corrected with glasses or medication. These devices are designed to enhance remaining vision and maximize functional vision. Examples of low-vision devices include magnifiers, telescopic lenses, electronic magnification systems, and video magnifiers. Low vision specialists can assess an individual's visual needs and recommend appropriate devices to aid reading, writing, or other daily activities.

- **Vision Rehabilitation:** Vision rehabilitation programs aim to help individuals with vision loss adapt to their visual impairment and maximize their independence. These programs, often delivered by occupational therapists or specialized vision rehabilitation professionals, provide training and strategies to develop alternative skills and techniques. They can include orientation and mobility training, activities of daily living (ADL) training, assistive technology instruction, and psychosocial support.

- **Surgical Interventions:** In some cases, surgical procedures may be an option to address specific eye conditions causing vision loss. Cataract surgery, for example, involves removing the clouded lens and replacing it with an artificial intraocular lens to restore vision. Some retinal conditions may require surgical interventions, such as retinal detachment repair or vitrectomy. It is essential to consult with an ophthalmologist to determine the suitability and potential benefits of surgical options.

- **Assistive Technology:** Advancements in technology have led to the development of various assistive devices that can support individuals with vision loss. Screen reading software, screen magnifiers, braille displays, and voice-activated systems are examples of assistive technology that can improve access to information, communication, and daily activities. Orientation and mobility apps, GPS navigation systems, and wearable devices can also assist with independent travel.

It is important to consult with an eye care professional, such as an ophthalmologist or optometrist, who specializes in managing vision loss. They can perform a comprehensive evaluation, provide a diagnosis, and recommend appropriate treatment options based on the specific needs and conditions of the individual. Additionally, vision rehabilitation specialists can offer guidance and support in adapting to vision loss and learning alternative techniques for daily living.

Taste and Smell Loss Treatments

Taste and smell loss, also known as anosmia and ageusia, can significantly affect a person's enjoyment of food, ability to detect odors, and overall quality of life. While complete recovery from these conditions may not always be possible, some treatments and interventions can help manage and potentially improve taste and smell loss. Here are some common approaches:

Identifying and Managing Underlying Causes

Various factors, including nasal congestion, respiratory infections, head injuries, certain medications, and neurological conditions, can cause loss of taste and smell. If possible, identifying and addressing the underlying cause is an essential step.

For example, treating nasal congestion with decongestants or addressing sinus infections can potentially improve smell and taste function. It is suggested that you consult with a healthcare professional to determine the cause and appropriate management strategies.

- *Medication Adjustment:* In cases where taste and smell loss are side effects of certain medications, adjusting the medication regimen or exploring alternative medications may be considered. However, this should only be done under the guidance of a healthcare professional, as medication adjustments should be carefully evaluated and monitored.

- *Smell Training:* Smell training involves repeated exposure to different scents to retrain the olfactory system and potentially improve smell function. This technique typically involves smelling essential oils or other strongly scented substances for a few minutes daily. By regularly exposing the olfactory system to these scents, some individuals have reported improvements in their ability to detect and identify odors. Smell training should be done under the guidance of a healthcare professional familiar with the technique.

- *Nutritional Counseling:* In cases where taste loss affects appetite or dietary habits, working with a registered dietitian or nutritionist can be helpful. They can provide guidance on optimizing nutrition, modifying food textures or flavors to compensate for taste loss, and ensuring a balanced and enjoyable diet.

- *Psychological Support:* Taste and smell loss can have a significant emotional impact on individuals, affecting their well-being and quality of life. Seeking psychological support, such as counseling or support groups, can provide a safe space to discuss and cope with the emotional aspects of these conditions. Support from others who have experienced similar challenges can be particularly beneficial.

It is important to note that the effectiveness of these treatments may vary depending on the underlying cause and the individual's specific situation. Additionally, for some individuals, taste and smell loss may be permanent or irreversible.

Suppose you are experiencing taste and smell loss. In that case, it is recommended to consult with a healthcare professional, such as an otolaryngologist (ear, nose, and throat specialist) or a neurologist, who can evaluate your condition, determine the underlying cause, and recommend appropriate treatment options or referrals to specialists in the field. They can provide personalized guidance and support based on your specific needs.

Touch and Tactile Loss Treatments

Touch and tactile loss can significantly impact an individual's ability to perceive and interact with their environment, affecting their overall quality of life. Fortunately, various treatments and interventions are available to address tactile loss and enhance tactile perception. These treatments aim to restore or improve the sense of touch, facilitating sensory experiences and supporting overall well-being. Here are some common touch and tactile loss treatments:

Tactile Stimulation and Sensory Integration

Tactile stimulation therapies involve engaging the sense of touch through various techniques, such as massage, pressure application, or texture exploration. These therapies aim to increase tactile awareness, improve sensory processing, and promote a positive sensory experience. Sensory integration techniques, often used in occupational therapy, focus on stimulating and integrating sensory input, including touch, and enhancing overall sensory function.

Assistive Devices

Assistive devices can play an important role in compensating for tactile loss. For example, tactile aids, such as textured gloves or sensory brushes, can provide additional tactile input and enhance the perception of touch. These devices can be particularly useful for individuals with limited tactile sensation or those who experience difficulties in processing tactile information.

- **Rehabilitation and Training Programs:** Rehabilitation programs designed for individuals with tactile loss can help improve tactile perception and sensory integration. These programs often involve structured activities and exercises to enhance sensory awareness, discrimination, and modulation. Occupational therapists, physical therapists, or specialized rehabilitation centers may provide these programs.
- **Virtual Reality (VR) and Haptic Technology:** Virtual reality (VR) technology, coupled with haptic

feedback, has shown promise in addressing tactile loss. VR environments can simulate different textures and sensations, allowing individuals to engage in virtual tactile experiences. Haptic technology provides touch-based feedback through specialized devices or gloves, enabling users to feel virtual objects and textures. These technologies offer opportunities for sensory retraining and the exploration of tactile sensations in a controlled and immersive environment.

- ***Neurorehabilitation and Neuroplasticity:*** The brain's remarkable capacity for neuroplasticity can be harnessed in neurorehabilitation programs. Through targeted therapies and exercises, individuals with tactile loss can stimulate neural pathways associated with touch, promoting the rewiring and reorganization of the brain to enhance tactile perception and integration.

It is important to note that the effectiveness of these treatments may vary depending on the underlying cause and severity of tactile loss. Therefore, a comprehensive assessment by a healthcare professional specializing in sensory disorders is key to determining the most appropriate treatment approach for each individual.

By addressing tactile loss and improving tactile perception, these treatments and interventions aim to enhance individuals' ability to engage with their environment, promote a sense of safety and well-being, and facilitate meaningful sensory experiences. They play a vital role in restoring the intricate connection between touch and our cognitive and emotional well-being.

Technological Advancements for Sensory Loss

In addition to conventional assistive technologies, alternative technologies are being developed to assist individuals with sensory loss. Here are a few examples:

- ***Virtual Reality (VR) and Augmented Reality (AR):*** VR and AR can simulate sensory experiences for individuals with sensory loss. For example, virtual reality environments can replicate visual or auditory stimuli to create immersive experiences for those with visual or hearing impairments. AR can overlay digital information onto the real world to enhance perception and provide context-aware assistance.

- *Brain-Computer Interfaces (BCIs):* BCIs establish a direct communication pathway between the brain and an external device without using the usual motor output pathways (e.g., muscles). BCIs can assist individuals with severe motor disabilities, allowing them to control devices or interact with the environment using their brain signals. BCIs hold potential for restoring sensory functions, such as vision or hearing, by directly stimulating the corresponding brain areas.
- *Electrocutaneous Stimulation:* Electrocutaneous stimulation involves electrical stimulation to provide sensory feedback to individuals with sensory loss. For example, in the case of vision loss, electrodes placed on the skin can stimulate the tactile sense to convey visual information. This approach is being explored to create sensory substitution devices that convert visual or auditory information into tactile sensations.
- *Assistive Wearable Devices:* Wearable devices, such as smart glasses or haptic feedback devices, can provide sensory feedback or augment sensory perception. For instance, wearable devices equipped with cameras and sensors can detect objects, obstacles, or faces and provide audio or tactile feedback to assist individuals with visual impairments.
- *Gene Therapy and Stem Cell Research:* Advancements in gene therapy and stem cell research hold promise for treating certain types of sensory loss. Researchers are exploring gene therapies to restore vision in individuals with genetic eye diseases, and stem cell research is being conducted to regenerate damaged auditory cells in cases of hearing loss.

It's important to note that many of these alternative technologies are still in the research and development stage, and their effectiveness and accessibility may vary. However, they demonstrate exciting possibilities for assisting individuals with sensory loss and improving their quality of life. Despite the current limitations, the rapid pace of innovation and the commitment of researchers and developers to address sensory deficits provide hope for more widespread and practical solutions in the near future, further enhancing the independence and well-being of those affected by sensory loss.

Medical Advancements

Medical advancements have significantly improved healthcare outcomes, enhanced patient care, and advanced our understanding of various medical conditions. Here are some notable medical advancements:

- **Precision Medicine:** Precision medicine considers individual variations in genes, environment, and lifestyle to tailor medical treatments and interventions. It enables personalized approaches to prevention, diagnosis, and treatment, leading to more effective and targeted healthcare.
- **Genomic Medicine:** The mapping of the human genome has paved the way for genomic medicine, which involves analyzing an individual's genetic information to understand their susceptibility to certain diseases and to develop personalized treatments. It has particularly influenced the fields of oncology, pharmacogenomics, and rare genetic disorders.
- **Immunotherapy and Targeted Therapies:** Immunotherapy has revolutionized cancer treatment by harnessing the body's immune system to fight cancer cells. Monoclonal antibodies, immune checkpoint inhibitors, and CAR-T cell therapy are examples of immunotherapies that have shown remarkable results in treating various types of cancer. Targeted therapies, which focus on specific molecular targets in cancer cells, have also emerged as effective treatment options.
- **Minimally Invasive Surgery:** Minimally invasive surgical techniques, such as laparoscopy and robotic surgery, have transformed the field of surgery. These procedures involve smaller incisions, reduced blood loss, faster recovery times, and fewer complications than traditional open surgeries.
- **Regenerative Medicine:** Regenerative medicine aims to replace or regenerate damaged tissues and organs using stem cells, tissue engineering, and biomaterials. It holds promise for treating conditions like organ failure, spinal cord injuries, and degenerative diseases.
- **Telemedicine and Remote Healthcare:** Telemedicine has expanded access to healthcare by enabling remote consultations, diagnosis, and monitoring. It has become

valuable in rural or underserved areas, allowing patients to receive medical care from a distance through video conferencing, remote monitoring devices, and mobile health applications.

- *Artificial Intelligence (AI) in Healthcare:* AI has the potential to transform healthcare by improving diagnostics, predicting disease outcomes, assisting in treatment planning, and enhancing patient care. AI algorithms can analyze vast medical data to provide insights and support clinical decision-making.

- *Advanced Imaging Technologies:* Medical imaging technologies, such as magnetic resonance imaging (MRI), computed tomography (CT), and positron emission tomography (PET), have undergone significant advancements. These technologies provide detailed images of the body's structures and functions, aiding in early detection, accurate diagnosis, and treatment planning.

These advancements represent just a fraction of the many breakthroughs and innovations that continue to shape the medical field. Ongoing research, technological developments, and interdisciplinary collaborations hold great promise for further advancements in healthcare.

Reflections on The Role of Vision, Hearing, Taste, Smell, and Touch in Memory

Our senses play a profound and intricate role in forming, retaining, and retrieving memories. From the sights we behold to the sounds we hear, the tastes we savor, the textures we feel, and the scents we inhale, each sensory experience leaves an indelible imprint on our memory tapestry.

Visual stimuli, such as stunning landscapes or vibrant hues, have the power to etch vivid images in our minds. They create mental snapshots that can transport us back to a specific moment, evoking emotions and enriching our recollection of past events. Audience cues, whether the melody of a familiar song or the sound of a loved one's voice, can trigger a cascade of memories, imbuing them with emotional resonance and lending a sense of familiarity.

Our sense of taste has an uncanny ability to evoke memories associated with specific flavors and culinary experiences. The mere taste of a dish can transport us back to cherished moments shared around the dinner table, reminding us of the people, places, and emotions intertwined with those sensory encounters.

Touch, too, leaves an enduring mark on our memory. The sensation of a gentle caress, the roughness of a textured surface, or the comforting embrace of a loved one can create lasting impressions that become woven into the fabric of our recollections. Whether it's the warmth of a summer breeze or the chill of snowflakes on our skin, tactile experiences can evoke tangible and emotionally charged.

And let us not forget the power of scent. The olfactory system possesses a unique ability to bypass rationality and directly tap into our emotional core. The aroma of freshly baked bread, the fragrance of blooming flowers, or the scent of a loved one's perfume can transport us back in time, triggering memories and emotions with astonishing clarity. Scent has an extraordinary capacity to evoke forgotten moments and breathe life into faded recollections.

CHAPTER 15

How Hormones Affect Memory

Hormones serve as the conductors in the complex orchestration of memory, influencing its formation and recall. Whether stress hormones, powerhouse hormones, or even blood sugar regulators like insulin, each hormone plays a unique role in the intricate dance of recollections. This behind-the-scenes hormonal choreography unveils the mysterious connections between physiology and memory.

The intricate interplay of hormones within the brain's symphony holds the key to optimal cognitive performance. Consider thyroid hormones as the maestros, expertly regulating weight and energy levels. The condition of hypothyroidism, characterized by an underactive thyroid, results in decreased energy, weight gain, and potential challenges to mental health, including depression and memory difficulties. Conversely, hyperthyroidism, caused by an overactive thyroid, is associated with weight loss, dry skin, and psychological changes, such as heightened anxiety and irritability.

Complementing the thyroid's influence, stress hormones like cortisol and adrenaline are pivotal in responding to life's challenges. They play an indispensable role in memory and cognition, potentially influencing concentration and contributing to the development of depression. Furthermore, sex hormones, notably estrogen and testosterone, extend their reach beyond reproductive functions, contributing significantly to cognitive health. These hormones influence memory and cognition, underscoring their significance in overall brain function. Growth hormones, often the unsung heroes, are integral to growth and metabolism, with subtle yet substantial impacts on cognitive performance. Imbalances in these hormones can lead to a range of cognitive challenges, affecting memory, attention, and overall mental well-being.

Lastly, the hormone oxytocin, commonly referred to as the "love hormone," plays a vital role in regulating social bonds, trust, and emotional regulation. It contributes to a nuanced emotional layer, influencing cognitive performance and psychological well-being.

Maintaining a delicate balance among thyroid hormones, stress hormones, sex hormones, growth hormones, and oxytocin is

133

indispensable to orchestrating optimal brain function. Imbalances in these hormones can lead to cognitive challenges, affecting memory, attention, and overall mental health. Acknowledging and appreciating the intricate role of hormones in cognitive intricacies is pivotal to understanding and optimizing brain function.

Hormone Imbalances and Memory Effects

Hormones are vital for regulating various bodily processes, including memory and cognitive function. When hormone levels are out of balance, it can affect our ability to focus, learn, and remember. Some hormones, like cortisol, estrogen, progesterone, and thyroid hormones, are particularly important for memory.

High levels of cortisol, a stress hormone, can make it harder to remember things. Too much cortisol can affect memory by interfering with the brain's ability to create and store new memories. Hormone levels in women can change during different life stages, like pregnancy or menopause. These hormonal fluctuations can impact memory. For example, some women may experience memory difficulties during menopause.

An imbalance in thyroid hormones can lead to cognitive issues. Both hypothyroidism (too little thyroid hormone) and hyperthyroidism (too much thyroid hormone) can affect memory and brain function. Hormone imbalances can affect memory differently from person to person. Factors like age, genetics, overall health, and lifestyle choices can influence how hormone imbalances impact memory.

Addressing hormone imbalances may require medical intervention and lifestyle modifications. Some options include hormone replacement therapy, dietary changes, stress management techniques, and regular exercise. It's important to understand the link between hormones and memory. Being aware of how hormones affect memory can help individuals recognize the potential impact of hormone imbalances on their mental well-being. Seeking appropriate interventions can help optimize cognitive performance. By maintaining a healthy balance of hormones, individuals can support their memory and overall brain health.

Thyroid Hormones

Thyroid hormones play an imperative role in regulating various bodily functions, including metabolism, growth, and development. They also have a significant impact on brain function and memory.

The two primary thyroid hormones, triiodothyronine (T3) and thyroxine (T4) are essential for maintaining cognitive health and supporting optimal memory performance.

Thyroid Hormones and Brain Function

Thyroid hormones are Important for brain development, particularly during infancy and childhood. They influence the growth and maturation of neurons, which are essential for memory formation and recall. In adults, thyroid hormones continue to support cognitive function by regulating neurotransmitter production and synaptic activity.

Thyroid hormones are vital for maintaining memory and cognitive function in adults. Deficiencies or excesses in thyroid hormone levels can lead to memory problems and cognitive impairment. For example, hypothyroidism, a condition characterized by low levels of thyroid hormones, can cause memory issues, slowed thinking, and difficulty concentrating.

Conversely, hyperthyroidism, a condition where thyroid hormone levels are too high, can also lead to memory problems, as well as other cognitive difficulties like anxiety and irritability.

Treatment for Thyroid-Related Memory Issues

Treatment for thyroid-related memory issues typically involves restoring thyroid hormone levels to a normal range. This can be achieved through medication, such as hormone replacement therapy, or by treating the underlying cause of the thyroid disorder. In some cases, lifestyle changes, such as improving diet and exercise habits, can also help improve memory and cognitive function.

In conclusion, Thyroid hormones play an essential role in regulating brain function and supporting memory performance. Imbalances in thyroid hormone levels can lead to memory problems and other cognitive difficulties. Early diagnosis and treatment of thyroid disorders can help restore normal hormone levels and improve memory and cognitive function. It's important to work closely with a healthcare provider to monitor thyroid hormone levels and manage any associated memory issues.

Stress Hormones

Chronic stress and prolonged exposure to stress hormones, such as cortisol and adrenaline, can have significant effects on memory, cognitive function, and physical health. Research has shown that glucocorticoids (GCs), the main class of stress hormones, are strongly linked to memory performance, and elevated GC levels are associated with memory performance decline in both normal and pathological aging.

Chronic stress and high levels of basal cortisol have been associated with impaired cognitive performance, decreased hippocampal volume, and increased risk of dementia and Alzheimer's disease. However, it's important to note that while cortisol can impair memory signals in the hippocampus as a whole, it also increases connectivity and enhances the brain's ability to encode memories.

Therefore, while acute stress can enhance memory encoding, chronic stress and prolonged exposure to stress hormones can have detrimental effects on memory, cognitive function, and physical health.

Stress and Memory

Stress hormones like cortisol are released in response to perceived threats or challenges. In the short term, these hormones can enhance memory and cognitive function by increasing alertness and attention. However, chronic exposure to stress hormones can have detrimental effects on memory, as prolonged elevation of cortisol levels may impair neural connections critical for efficient information processing and retention.

Chronic Stress and Memory

Chronic stress, marked by persistent activation of the body's stress response system, can impair memory and cognitive function. High levels of cortisol can disrupt the brain's ability to consolidate and retrieve memories, leading to difficulties with both short-term and long-term memory. This sustained stress response may also contribute to a decline in overall mental well-being over time.

Stress and Working Memory

Working memory, which refers to the ability to hold and manipulate information in the mind over short periods, is particularly vulnerable to the effects of stress. Chronic stress can impair working memory, making it more difficult to focus, concentrate, and perform complex tasks.

Stress and Episodic Memory

Episodic memory, which involves the recollection of specific experiences or events, can also be affected by stress. Chronic stress can impair the consolidation and retrieval of episodic memories, leading to difficulties in remembering specific events and experiences.

Managing Stress to Improve Memory

Managing stress is key to maintaining optimal memory and cognitive function. Effective stress management techniques include regular exercise, mindfulness meditation, and engaging in stress-reducing activities like yoga or deep breathing exercises. In some cases, therapy or counseling may also be helpful in managing stress and improving memory.

In conclusion, stress hormones like cortisol and adrenaline play an important role in regulating the body's response to stress. However, chronic stress and prolonged exposure to stress hormones can impair memory and cognitive function. Effective stress management techniques, such as exercise, meditation, and therapy, can help mitigate the negative effects of stress on memory and cognitive function, promoting overall mental well-being.

Sex Hormones

Sex hormones, including estrogen, testosterone, and progesterone, play a crucial role in cognitive function and memory. Their effects can vary depending on gender, age, and overall health. Understanding the intricate relationship between sex hormones and memory is important for maintaining optimal cognitive health and well-being.

Estrogen

Estrogen, the primary female sex hormone, is vital for cognitive function and memory, particularly in women. Estrogen receptors are found throughout the brain, including areas involved in learning and memory, such as the hippocampus.

Estrogen has been shown to promote the growth of new neurons and enhance synaptic plasticity, which is essential for memory formation and consolidation.

During menopause, when estrogen levels decline, some women may experience memory difficulties and cognitive impairment. Estrogen therapy has been found to improve memory and cognitive function in postmenopausal women. In addition, research suggests that estrogen may help protect against neurodegenerative diseases, such as Alzheimer's disease, by reducing inflammation and promoting neuronal health.

Testosterone

Testosterone, the primary male sex hormone, also plays a role in cognitive function and memory, particularly in men. Testosterone receptors are found in brain areas involved in memory and learning, such as the hippocampus and prefrontal cortex. Testosterone has been shown to enhance memory consolidation and retrieval, particularly for spatial memory tasks.

Low testosterone levels have been associated with memory problems and cognitive decline in men. Testosterone therapy has been found to improve memory and cognitive function in men with low testosterone levels.

However, it is important to note that testosterone therapy can have potential side effects, including an increased risk of blood clots and cardiovascular issues. Therefore, it is important to work with a healthcare provider to determine if testosterone therapy is appropriate and to monitor its effects.

Progesterone

Progesterone, another female sex hormone, has also been associated with cognitive function and memory. Progesterone has neuroprotective effects and has been shown to promote neuronal growth and differentiation.

Some research suggests that progesterone may enhance memory consolidation and retrieval, particularly for spatial memory tasks. Progesterone levels fluctuate throughout the menstrual cycle and decrease during menopause.

Some studies have found that progesterone levels are associated with better memory and overall cognition in women, particularly in the early stages of menopause. However, more research is needed to fully understand the relationship between progesterone and memory.

In conclusion, Sex hormones play an indispensable role in cognitive function and memory. Estrogen, testosterone, and progesterone all have distinct effects on cognitive function and memory, with their influence varying depending on gender, age, and overall health. Understanding the intricate relationship between sex hormones and memory is important for maintaining optimal cognitive health and well-being.

Growth Hormones

Growth hormones, such as human growth hormone (HGH) and insulin-like growth factor-1 (IGF-1), have been linked to cognitive function and memory. Growth hormones are secreted by the pituitary gland and play a key role in growth, metabolism, and tissue repair. They also have an impact on brain function and cognitive performance.

Growth Hormones and Cognitive Function

Growth hormones have been shown to enhance cognitive function, including memory, learning, and attention. They promote neuronal growth and differentiation, enhance synaptic plasticity, and promote the formation of new neurons in the brain. Growth hormones may also protect neurons from damage and promote neuronal survival, which is important for maintaining cognitive function and memory.

Growth Hormones and Memory Formation

Growth hormones have been found to enhance memory formation and consolidation. They promote the release of neurotransmitters, such as acetylcholine and glutamate, which are essential for memory formation. Growth hormones may also enhance the activity of enzymes involved in memory formation, such as protein kinase C and calcium/calmodulin-dependent protein kinase II.

Growth Hormone Deficiency and Memory

Growth hormone deficiency, which can occur due to pituitary gland disorders or aging, has been linked to cognitive decline and memory impairment. Studies have shown that individuals with growth hormone deficiency have poorer memory and cognitive function compared to healthy individuals. Growth hormone therapy has been shown to improve memory and cognitive function in individuals with growth hormone deficiency.

Growth hormones may also enhance memory formation and consolidation. Growth hormone deficiency has been linked to cognitive decline and memory impairment, but growth hormone therapy has been shown to improve memory and cognitive function in individuals with growth hormone deficiency. Understanding the relationship between growth hormones and memory is important for maintaining optimal cognitive health and well-being.

Oxytocin

Oxytocin, the "love hormone," has multifaceted effects on memory that extend far beyond social contexts and into therapeutic considerations. Its impact on memory processes is influenced by a myriad of factors, such as social contexts, selective amnesic effects, intrusive memories, memory enhancement, potential therapeutic roles, modulation of memory recall, and even its role in diseases like Alzheimer's.

While oxytocin has been found to cause memory impairment and amnesic effects in humans, it can also strengthen or weaken performance on memory tasks depending on the individual's personality traits and the specific context. This complexity underscores the intricate relationship between oxytocin and memory formation, consolidation, and retrieval.

Interestingly, research has shown that oxytocin can also strengthen negative social memories and contribute to future anxiety, which may have significant implications for conditions such as post-traumatic stress disorder (PTSD). This finding highlights the potential therapeutic applications of oxytocin in modulating traumatic memories and alleviating associated psychological distress.

However, the impact of oxytocin on memory is multidimensional and not fully understood, as its effects can vary based on factors like dosage, timing of administration, and individual differences in neurophysiology and psychology. Ongoing research continues to unravel the nuances of oxytocin's role in memory processes, paving the way for potential therapeutic interventions and a deeper understanding of the intricate interplay between hormones, emotions, and cognitive functions.

Oxytocin and Memory Encoding

The influence of social contexts on oxytocin's effects on memory encoding highlights the interconnectedness of social factors and cognitive processes. Oxytocin enhances memory for socially relevant information, particularly in comfortable and trusting social situations. Oxytocin's effects on memory encoding are influenced by social engagement and active participation, as well as the emotional significance of social interactions. Understanding this interconnectedness allows us to improve memory function, whether for academic achievement, professional success, or enriching personal relationships.

Selective Amnesic Effects of Oxytocin

Oxytocin has been found to exhibit selective amnesic effects on human memory. The type of memory can influence oxytocin's impact, emphasizing its nuanced role in memory processes. This suggests that oxytocin may have specific effects on certain types of memories.

Oxytocin and Intrusive Memories

Oxytocin administration during trauma analogs may increase intrusive memories, which are core symptoms of post-traumatic experiences. This suggests that oxytocin may have a role in regulating memories of traumatic events.

Oxytocin and Memory Performance

Studies demonstrate that oxytocin can enhance social memory in rodents, promote rapid adaptation to fear signals in social contexts and facilitate memory processes. This suggests that oxytocin may play an important role in the formation and consolidation of memories.

Oxytocin and Alzheimer's Disease

Oxytocin's ability to strengthen social memory and improve spatial memory raises the question of its potential therapeutic role in conditions like Alzheimer's disease. This suggests that oxytocin may be a promising avenue for the treatment of memory impairments associated with neurodegenerative diseases.

Oxytocin and Modulation of Memory Recall

Intranasal oxytocin, compared to placebo, may influence memory recall. It has been found to decrease the number of over-general memories recalled while increasing the recall of specific memories. This suggests that oxytocin may modulate the recall of different types of memories.

In conclusion, oxytocin's intricate influence on memory processes underscores its role not only in social contexts but also in therapeutic considerations for conditions involving memory impairments. Further research is needed to fully understand the complex relationship between oxytocin and memory and to explore its potential therapeutic applications.

Reflections on How Hormones Affect Memory

The realm of hormones, where these intricate messengers orchestrate a symphony of physiological processes and exert a profound influence on our memory functions. It's truly captivating how this interplay between our physical selves and the cognitive mechanisms that shape our memories unfolds.

When stress knocks on our door, our cortisol levels surge like a tidal wave, impacting a crucial brain region known as the hippocampus. This hormonal upheaval can disrupt the formation and retrieval of memories, resulting in hazy and less accurate recollections. Imagine standing on the shore of your memories, watching as the waves of cortisol crash against the shores of your hippocampus, leaving a temporary haze in their wake. It's as if the stress-induced storm disrupts the calm waters of memory, making it harder to navigate and retrieve the information we seek.

Reproductive hormones such as estrogen and progesterone also leave their imprint on memory performance. These hormones, with their ebb and flow throughout the menstrual cycle, showcase the nuanced role of hormonal fluctuations in cognitive processes. During certain phases, estrogen levels rise, enhancing memory formation and recall. In contrast, progesterone can have a more inhibitory effect on memory, leading to temporary lapses in retrieval. It's as if the hormonal symphony of our reproductive system conducts a delicate dance, influencing the tempo and rhythm of our memory abilities.

Let's not forget about the thyroid hormones, those regulators of metabolism that also play a significant role in memory function. These hormones, in their delicate balance, influence the consolidation and retrieval of memories. When thyroid hormone levels are out of balance, conditions such as hypothyroidism or hyperthyroidism can significantly impact memory and cognition. It's as if the thyroid hormones are the conductors of our metabolic orchestra, ensuring that the energy and resources necessary for memory processes are in perfect harmony.

However, hormones do not act alone in this grand performance. They collaborate with neurotransmitters, the messengers of the mind, to orchestrate the intricate dance of memory formation and recall. Influenced by hormones, neurotransmitters like serotonin and dopamine regulate our moods and imbue our memories with emotional hues. It's as if the hormones and neurotransmitters are partners in a breathtaking tango, guiding the steps of memory formation and recall. The delicate interplay between hormones, neurotransmitters, and the essence of our memories illustrates the intricate and dynamic nature of the mind-body connection.

CHAPTER 16

The Effect of Brain Injury on Memory and Learning

Exploring the aftermath of brain injury unveils the remarkable resilience of the human brain. In this dynamic narrative, the brain, akin to a skilled artisan, strives to rewire its neural pathways, demonstrating extraordinary adaptability in the face of adversity. This story transcends setbacks, highlighting resilience as the hero in the intricate dance between trauma and recovery within the complex terrain of memory and learning.

Imagine the mind as a bustling cityscape, a vibrant tapestry woven with memories and thoughts. Suddenly, a storm rips through, a traumatic brain injury or an acquired one – a violent blow, a silent stroke, a seemingly harmless tumble. The streets crack, buildings crumble, and the once-familiar landscape transforms into a maze of confusion and frustration.

This is the harsh reality for many facing the aftermath of such storms. The storm doesn't just leave wounds visible on the outside; it scars the very tapestry of memory. Faces blur, conversations fade, and the once-automaticity of daily routines becomes a frustrating puzzle. The storm disrupts attention and focus, flickering like dying streetlights. Even language, the bridge between minds, can collapse, leaving individuals struggling to speak or understand.

But understanding these storms and their paths through the cityscape of the mind is the key to rebuilding. Careful scans paint a grim picture of the devastation, like aerial maps of the ravaged city. Neurologists, therapists, and other specialists – akin to architects and engineers – come together to map a path to recovery.

The road back is long and arduous, each brick of cognitive skill painstakingly laid. Therapists become memory trainers, teaching the reweaving of faded tapestries. Attention is coaxed back, like tending a dying flame. Language, the fallen bridge, is painstakingly rebuilt word by word.

It's a battle hard-fought, a journey riddled with setbacks and stumbles. But hope remains, a beacon even in the storm's aftermath. Because the mind, like a resilient city, has the power to rebuild. With support, research, and unwavering determination, individuals can reclaim their streets, brick by memory brick, thought by thought. By understanding the storms that scar the mind, we can become helping hands, rebuilding individual lives and collective resilience in the face of the most complex challenges.

Understanding how TBIs and acquired brain injuries impact memory and cognition is critical for effective diagnosis, treatment, and rehabilitation.

Episodic Memory Impairments

One of the hallmark consequences of TBIs and acquired brain injuries is the disruption of episodic memory processes. Episodic memory refers to remembering specific events, experiences, and personal narratives. Individuals with these injuries often experience difficulties in various aspects of episodic memory, including:

- **Recall:** The ability to intentionally retrieve specific details or events from the past is frequently impaired. This can manifest as forgetfulness about recent or past events.
- **Recognition:** Recognizing previously encountered information or people may be compromised. Individuals might have difficulty identifying familiar faces or objects.
- **Visual Memory:** Visual memory deficits can affect an individual's ability to remember and navigate through familiar environments. Tasks like recognizing landmarks or following directions may become challenging.
- **Verbal Memory:** The capacity to recall spoken or written information can be impaired, leading to difficulties in understanding and communicating.
- **Immediate and Delayed Effects:** TBIs often lead to rapid memory disruptions following the injury. However, some individuals may also experience delayed memory problems that emerge days or weeks after the injury. This delayed onset of memory difficulties underscores the need for ongoing monitoring and rehabilitation.

The profound disruptions in episodic memory processes resulting from TBIs and acquired brain injuries intricately affect various dimensions of an individual's cognitive functioning. For those navigating the complexities of these injuries, the journey involves addressing the immediate impact and recognizing the potential for delayed onset memory problems.

In a clinical setting, a multidisciplinary team, including neurologists, neurosurgeons, radiologists, neuropsychologists, and rehabilitation therapists, often collaborates to provide a comprehensive assessment and treatment plan for a person with a TBI.

Diagnostic Evaluation

A diagnostic evaluation for a traumatic brain injury (TBI) involves several steps and tools to assess the extent and impact of the injury. The goal is to determine the severity of the trauma, the specific brain regions affected, and the implications for the patient's cognitive, physical, and emotional functioning. Here is a structured breakdown of the process:

- *Quality of Life:* Episodic memory is fundamental to our ability to recall personal experiences and events. Impairments in this memory type can significantly impact an individual's quality of life, hindering their capacity to reminisce about meaningful moments and engage in everyday activities.
- *Functional Independence:* Episodic memory plays a pivotal role in maintaining functional independence. Individuals with impairments may struggle with routine tasks, such as remembering appointments, following instructions, or navigating familiar environments, affecting their autonomy.
- *Diagnostic Insight:* Episodic memory assessments serve as valuable diagnostic tools, aiding healthcare professionals in identifying and understanding the extent of brain injuries, including traumatic brain injuries (TBIs). Accurate diagnosis is essential for appropriate treatment planning and interventions.
- *Research Advancements:* Research into episodic memory impairments advances our understanding of brain function and cognitive processes. This knowledge is essential for developing targeted therapies, interventions, and rehabilitation strategies to mitigate the impact of memory deficits.
- *Rehabilitation Strategies:* Determining episodic memory impairments informs the development of tailored rehabilitation programs. These programs aim to enhance memory function, promote cognitive resilience, and

THE TAPESTRY OF MEMORY: UNRAVELING THE THREADS OF THE MIND

facilitate the reintegration of individuals into their communities.

- **Psychosocial Well-being:** Memory is intricately linked to personal identity and relationships. Episodic memory impairments can strain social connections and contribute to emotional challenges. Recognizing and addressing these impairments is essential for supporting the psychosocial well-being of affected individuals.

Determining episodic memory impairments is vital for personalized care, effective rehabilitation, and advancements in our understanding of cognitive function, ultimately contributing to improved outcomes and the overall well-being of individuals with such impairments.

The Diagnostic Evaluation Steps

A diagnostic evaluation for a traumatic brain injury (TBI) involves several steps and tools to assess the extent and impact of the injury. The goal is to determine the severity of the trauma, the specific brain regions affected, and the implications for the patient's cognitive, physical, and emotional functioning. Here is a structured breakdown of the process:

Medical Evaluation

The first step is a thorough medical history and symptom evaluation. This includes details about the injury itself, any loss of consciousness, current symptoms (headache, dizziness, memory problems, etc.), and any pre-existing medical conditions.

Neurological Examination

A neurological examination is a systematic assessment a healthcare provider performs to evaluate the nervous system's function. It includes a series of tests and observations to assess the brain, spinal cord, and the network of nerves that link these organs to the rest of the body. The examination is designed to identify signs of neurological disorder or injury and helps diagnose conditions that affect the nervous system. Here are the key components of a neurological examination:

- **Mental Status:** In the context of a traumatic brain injury (TBI), a mental state evaluation is like stepping into a detective's shoes. It's a meticulous investigation, piecing together clues scattered across the landscape of someone's mind after the storm of a TBI. This evaluation isn't a cold interrogation; it's a compassionate conversation, a careful observation, and a gentle exploration of thoughts, emotions, and behaviors. A mental status evaluation includes the following:

- **Consciousness:** Assessing the patient's level of alertness and orientation to time, place, and person.
- **Attention and Concentration:** Testing the ability to focus and maintain attention.
- **Memory:** Testing both short-term and long-term memory recall.
- Language: Assessing speech for fluency, comprehension, and ability to name objects.
- **Higher Cognitive Functions:** Tasks to evaluate reasoning, problem-solving, and executive functions.

Cranial Nerves

The cranial nerves are a special set of twelve pairs of nerves that originate directly from the brain, unlike other nerves that emerge from the spinal cord. They play a vital role in connecting your brain to various parts of your head, neck, and even some upper body organs, managing sensory input and motor output.

Examining cranial nerve function reveals potential functional impairments caused by the TBI, such as impaired vision, facial movement, or swallowing. This can significantly impact daily living and require targeted rehabilitation interventions.

Motor System

After a brain injury, testing the motor system isn't just about flexing muscles. It's a vital tool that maps the damage, identifies daily struggles, guides recovery, and predicts long-term potential. This hidden conversation with the body helps rebuild movement, independence, and hope, one step at a time. A motor system test includes the following:

- **Muscle Strength:** Testing major muscle groups for strength.
- **Muscle Tone**: Assessing the resistance of muscles to passive movement.
- **Coordination and Fine Movements:** Performing tasks like finger-to-nose or heel-to-shin tests.
- **Involuntary Movements:** Observing for tremors, tics, or other abnormal movements.

Reflexes

Reflex tests after brain injuries are like deciphering Morse code from the nervous system. They map damage, reveal hidden struggles, guide recovery, and even predict the future. Following a traumatic brain injury (TBI), assessing neural connectivity becomes key in charting the path to recovery. Reflexes, those seemingly simple twitches, offer a potent window into the integrity of corticospinal and brainstem circuitry. A reflex test includes:

1. **Deep Tendon Reflexes:** Using a reflex hammer to check responses, such as the knee-jerk reflex.
2. **Superficial Reflexes:** Responses like the abdominal reflex or plantar reflex (Babinski sign).
3. **Pathological Reflexes:** These are reflexes that typically are not present in healthy adults and can indicate neurological problems.

Sensory System

The sensory system is the orchestra conductor of our experience, harmonizing sight, sound, touch, taste, smell, and even balance to paint a vibrant picture of the world around us. Think of it like fixing a puzzle. Each test is a piece, showing where the wires got crossed in your brain. With enough pieces, doctors can figure out how to put everything back together. The most common sensory tests include:

- **Sight:** Clarity of distant vision, ability to see close objects, mapping the visual field to detect blind spots or abnormalities, identifying numbers within colored circles to measure color perception, and distinguishing between light and dark.
- **Sound:** Measuring hearing thresholds for different frequencies, understanding spoken words in background noise, identifying the direction of sound source, and interpreting sounds and music.
- **Smell:** Pinpointing common scents like sweet, salty, sour, bitter, and umami, increasing and decreasing the concentration of an odorant to gauge the sensitivity of olfactory receptors and the brain's ability to bind olfactory cues with memories and emotions.
- **Taste:** Identifying five basic tastes, the sensitivity of taste buds, and differentiating complex flavor profiles.
- **Touch:** Testing sensitivity to light pressure on the skin, identifying pinpricks, hot and cold stimuli, feeling a tuning

fork placed on the body, and recognizing objects by touch without visual cues.

- *Gait and Stance:* Walking patterns, balance, and coordination. Regularity in steps, evaluating balance while standing still, identifying abnormalities in balance with eyes open and closed, and walking patterns for dynamic balance.

Autonomic Function

Assessing functions controlled by the autonomic nervous system, such as heart rate, blood pressure, sweating, and bowel and bladder control.

The findings from a neurological examination, when combined with the patient's history and other diagnostic tests (e.g., imaging, blood tests), help to guide further evaluation, diagnosis, and treatment planning for a variety of neurological conditions, including traumatic brain injury, stroke, multiple sclerosis, and epilepsy, to name a few.

Neuropsychological Testing

Neuropsychological testing is a comprehensive assessment method used to evaluate cognitive, emotional, and behavioral functions associated with brain function. These tests measure various cognitive domains, including memory, attention, language, executive functions, and visuospatial skills. Neuropsychological testing involves standardized tests, questionnaires, and interviews, providing valuable insights into an individual's cognitive abilities. Neuropsychological tests include:

- *Cognitive Tests:* These tests assess various cognitive domains like memory, attention, concentration, problem-solving, and executive function. Standard tests include the Wechsler Adult Intelligence Scale (WAIS), which assesses overall cognitive abilities; the Trail Making Test, which evaluates attention and processing speed; and the Rey Auditory Verbal Learning Test (RAVLT), which assesses memory.
- *Behavioral Tests:* These tests evaluate emotional and behavioral changes that might be associated with TBI, such as depression, anxiety, and impulsivity. Some commonly used tests include The Beck Depression Inventory (BDI), which measures depression symptoms, while the State-Trait Anxiety Inventory (STAI) assesses anxiety levels. The

Barratt Impulsiveness Scale (BIS) gauges impulsivity. These tools help clinicians understand and address psychological concerns effectively.

Additional Tests

- *Electroencephalogram (EEG):* measures electrical activity in the brain and can help identify seizures or other brain abnormalities.
- *Blood test:* It may be ordered to check for blood markers associated with TBI or to rule out other medical conditions.

It's important to remember that the specific diagnostic approach may vary depending on the severity of the TBI and the individual's symptoms. A team of healthcare professionals, including neurologists, neuropsychologists, and rehabilitation specialists, may be involved in the diagnostic process.

Treatment and Rehabilitation

Early intervention is critical to maximizing recovery and restoring cognitive function. Rehabilitation programs, including cognitive, physical, and occupational therapy, address memory deficits, improve cognitive skills, and enhance overall well-being.

Treatment and rehabilitation after a Traumatic Brain Injury (TBI) typically involve a multi-disciplinary approach to address physical, cognitive, and emotional challenges. The specific steps may vary based on the severity of the injury but commonly include the following:

- *Medical Stabilization:* Immediate medical attention to address life-threatening conditions and ensure stabilization.
- *Neurosurgical Intervention:* Surgery may be required for some instances, such as removing hematomas or repairing skull fractures.
- *Acute Medical Care:* Monitoring and managing complications, preventing secondary injuries, and addressing medical needs.
- *Rehabilitation Assessment:* Comprehensive evaluation by a rehabilitation team to assess cognitive, physical, and emotional impairments.
- *Physical Therapy:* Focuses on improving mobility, strength, balance, and coordination.

- *Occupational Therapy:* Helps individuals regain independence in daily activities and enhance cognitive skills.
- *Speech-Language Therapy:* Addresses communication and swallowing difficulties, common after a TBI.
- *Cognitive Rehabilitation:* Targets cognitive impairments through exercises and strategies to improve memory, attention, and executive functions.
- *Psychological Support:* Counseling and psychotherapy to address emotional and psychological challenges associated with the TBI.
- *Medication Management:* Prescription of medications to manage symptoms like pain, seizures, or mood disorders.
- *Community Reintegration:* Transitioning back into the community with support, focusing on social, vocational, and educational goals.
- *Follow-up Care:* Ongoing medical and rehabilitation follow-ups to monitor progress and address evolving needs.
- *Supportive Services:* Accessing support groups, vocational rehabilitation, and community resources to enhance overall well-being.
- *Long-Term Monitoring:* Periodic assessments to monitor any lingering effects or emerging issues and adjust interventions accordingly.

The specific plan is tailored to the individual's needs and may involve collaboration between neurologists, physiatrists, neuropsychologists, therapists, and other healthcare professionals. Rehabilitation is often a gradual process, and the goal is to maximize independence and quality of life for individuals recovering from a TBI.

TBIs and acquired brain injuries can have profound and lasting effects on memory and cognition. However, with the proper diagnosis, treatment, and rehabilitation, individuals can make significant strides in regaining cognitive function and improving their quality of life. The journey toward recovery is often a collaborative effort involving healthcare professionals, rehabilitation specialists, and a strong support network, all working together to help individuals rebuild their cognitive abilities and move forward with resilience and hope.

Reflections on The Effect of Brain Injury on Memory and Learning

We embark on a captivating expedition to delve into the intricate dynamics of how injuries to the brain profoundly shape our ability to recall memories and acquire new knowledge. Imagine this journey as an intellectual adventure, reminiscent of solving a captivating mystery – a quest to fathom how bumps, jolts, or injuries to the brain intricately influence our memory retention and learning capacities.

Instead of wading through dense scientific terminology, envision this exploration as a practical endeavor aimed at grasping the palpable impact of brain injuries on our cognitive processes. We're not immersing ourselves in the complexities of advanced scientific jargon; rather, we're adopting a straightforward approach to understanding how brain injuries might disrupt our memory recall and learning capabilities.

In this intellectual odyssey, we're not venturing into the realm of lofty scientific discourse; we're simply striving to comprehend how these injuries can potentially interfere with our memory and learning mechanisms. Picture it as an engaging puzzle-solving experience, where we connect the dots between a brain injury and the nuances of what we remember or find challenging to learn. It's an expedition of discovery, a hands-on effort to demystify the impact of brain injuries on the fundamental aspects of memory and learning. Prepare for an enlightening journey into the intersection of brain injuries, memory, and the acquisition of knowledge.

CHAPTER 17

The Role of Toxins in Memory Loss

Our remarkable brains, orchestrators of our memories, are susceptible to environmental toxins, disrupting the delicate balance pivotal for memory function. Unraveling this connection is like deciphering a cryptic code, offering profound insights into how external factors impact our cognitive landscape. This understanding becomes a call to action—a chance to safeguard our physical health and the symphony of memories in the grand theater of our minds.

Environmental toxins have been increasingly recognized for their potential role in memory loss and cognitive decline. The connection between exposure to these toxins and adverse effects on cognitive function is a growing concern in scientific research.

The intricate link between the environment and memory health has captured the attention of scientists and the public alike, highlighting the need to better understand the impact of toxic metals, pesticides, and industrial chemicals on our cognitive functions. This fascinating area of research underscores the intricate relationship between our surroundings and our mental well-being. The complex interplay between environmental contaminants and memory has become a pressing concern, emphasizing the importance of exploring the complex interconnections between these factors to identify potential strategies to safeguard memory health and optimize cognitive function.

Diving deeper into this intricate web of factors offers a unique opportunity to uncover new insights into the mechanisms underlying memory impairment and to discover novel strategies for promoting memory health and cognitive well-being. By unraveling the intricate dance between environmental toxins and memory, we can better understand how our environment impacts our cognitive function and develop effective interventions to protect our mental health. This fascinating journey of discovery invites us to explore the intricate relationship between the world around us and the health of our minds, shedding light on the intricate tapestry of factors that shape our cognitive landscape, which is essential for public health awareness and preventive measures.

In this chapter, we discover the intricate relationship between environmental toxins and memory loss, aiming to shed light on the mechanisms through which these toxins influence cognitive function.

Environmental Contaminants and Memory Loss

Numerous studies have established a compelling link between exposure to these substances and the profound impact they can have on memory. As we navigate through the intricate web of scientific findings, it becomes evident that such contaminants in our surroundings pose a tangible threat to our cognitive well-being.

The exploration of these connection sheds light on the potential dangers. It underscores the pressing need for a deeper understanding of how environmental factors contribute to memory loss and cognitive decline. Let's delve into the intricate relationship between environmental contaminants and cognitive function, focusing on toxic metals, pesticides, and industrial chemicals.

Toxic Metals

Toxic metals, such as lead, mercury, and cadmium, have been linked to memory impairment. Lead exposure, often associated with old paint and pipes, can interfere with memory formation and retrieval. Mercury, commonly found in fish and dental fillings, has also been associated with memory problems. Cadmium, found in cigarette smoke and industrial processes, can impair memory and cognitive function. Understanding the mechanisms by which these metals affect memory and developing strategies to reduce exposure is Important for safeguarding memory health.

Pesticides

Pesticides, such as organophosphates and pyrethroids, have been linked to memory impairment. Organophosphates, commonly used in agriculture, can interfere with memory processes. Pyrethroids, often used in homes and gardens, have been associated with memory problems. Research on the effects of pesticides on memory and strategies for reducing exposure is essential for protecting memory health.

Industrial Chemicals

Industrial chemicals, such as polychlorinated biphenyls (PCBs) and perfluoroalkyl substances (PFAS), have been linked to memory impairment. PCBs, found in electrical transformers and capacitors, can impair memory and cognitive function. PFAS, found in non-stick cookware and fire-fighting foams, can interfere with memory processes. Exploring the mechanisms by which these chemicals affect memory and developing strategies to reduce exposure is indispensable for safeguarding memory health.

Exposure to toxic metals, pesticides, and industrial chemicals can harm memory and cognitive function through various mechanisms, including neurotoxicity, chemical interference, oxidative stress, inflammation, structural changes, neurotransmitter imbalance, and impaired synaptic function. Understanding the specific toxins involved and their mechanisms of action is imperative for assessing and addressing memory problems resulting from toxin exposure. Minimizing exposure to environmental toxins and advocating for environmental regulations can help protect cognitive health.

Understanding Brain Toxicity

Neurotoxicology is the study of toxins' effects on the nervous system, particularly the brain, leading to adverse neurological outcomes, including memory loss and cognitive impairment. Certain toxins directly damage neurons, disrupting communication between brain cells and impacting cognitive processes. Acute toxic encephalopathies, characterized by sudden severe brain dysfunction due to toxic substances, can induce cognitive impairments, including memory problems.

Toxins in acute encephalopathies interfere with memory formation, induce oxidative stress, trigger inflammation, and alter synaptic function, contributing to memory deficits. The impact on cognitive function may be temporary or permanent, influenced by exposure duration, severity, and individual susceptibility.

Toxic encephalopathies manifest with various symptoms:

- **Confusion:** Toxic encephalopathies can lead to a state of mental disorientation, where individuals may struggle to comprehend their surroundings, experience memory lapses, or exhibit general cognitive bewilderment.
- **Difficulty Concentrating:** Impaired focus and attention are common symptoms, making it challenging for individuals to concentrate on tasks, follow

conversations, or maintain sustained attention on specific activities.

- **Impaired Judgment:** Toxic encephalopathies may compromise one's ability to make sound decisions and assess situations accurately. This can result in risky behaviors or poor decision-making.
- **Seizures:** A more severe manifestation, toxic encephalopathies can induce abnormal electrical activity in the brain, leading to seizures. These seizures may vary in intensity and duration, further contributing to the complexity of the neurological symptoms.

Timely identification and treatment of toxin exposure are Important to minimize long-term cognitive consequences. This involves removing the individual from the toxin source, providing supportive care, and administering specific treatments depending on the toxin involved.

In summary, neurotoxicology's significance lies in understanding the link between toxin exposure and memory loss. Acute toxic encephalopathies, with their severe impact on cognitive function, necessitate prompt identification and management to mitigate potential long-term consequences on cognitive function and promote optimal recovery.

Types of Neurotoxins and Intoxications

Naturally occurring neurotoxins are substances that are found in nature and can have toxic effects on the nervous system. For example, certain plants and fungi produce neurotoxins as a defense mechanism against predators. These neurotoxins can interfere with synaptic function, disrupt neurotransmitter systems, and damage neurons, ultimately impacting cognitive processes such as memory.

On the other hand, neurotoxins produced by human activities are substances that are synthesized or released as a result of human actions. These include industrial chemicals, pesticides, heavy metals, air pollutants, and recreational drugs. Human-produced neurotoxins can enter the environment through various means, such as pollution, occupational exposure, or substance abuse.

Both naturally occurring and human-produced neurotoxins can disrupt the mammalian nervous system in several ways. They can directly damage neurons, impair synaptic function, interfere with neurotransmitter systems, induce oxidative stress, trigger inflammation, and lead to structural changes in the brain. These disruptions can hinder the formation of new memories, impair the retrieval of existing memories, and impact cognitive function overall.

The specific effects of neurotoxins on memory can vary depending on the type of toxin and the extent of exposure. For example, pesticide exposure has been linked to cognitive impairment, while certain industrial chemicals can affect working memory. Additionally, substances like alcohol and recreational drugs can cause temporary memory blackouts.

It is important to note that the impact of neurotoxins on memory can vary among individuals. Factors such as genetics, duration of exposure, toxin dosage, and overall health can influence the extent of cognitive impairment. Furthermore, the long-term consequences of toxin exposure on memory can be significant, especially if the exposure is chronic or occurs during indispensable periods of brain development.

Understanding the different types of neurotoxins and their mechanisms of action is key for assessing and addressing memory problems resulting from toxin exposure. Minimizing toxin exposure through adopting a healthy lifestyle, reducing occupational hazards, and advocating for environmental regulations can help protect cognitive health. Seeking medical attention in cases of known or suspected toxin exposure is also important for preserving cognitive function and memory.

Mechanisms of Toxin-Induced Cognitive Impairment

Toxins can have detrimental effects on cognitive function, including learning and memory processes. Several mechanisms that contribute to toxin-induced cognitive impairment have been identified. Here, we will review some of these mechanisms and explore how toxins affect learning and memory.

- *Neurotransmission and synaptic plasticity impairment:* Toxins can disrupt neurotransmission, which is essential for proper communication between neurons. For example, lead exposure has been shown to interfere with the NMDA receptor, a key receptor involved in synaptic plasticity learning and memory. Toxins can also alter the release of neurotransmitters such as glutamate and GABA, affecting synaptic transmission.
- *Oxidative stress:* Many toxins induce oxidative stress, which occurs when there is an imbalance between the

production of reactive oxygen species (ROS) and the body's antioxidant defenses. Oxidative stress can lead to damage to neurons and impair cognitive function. Mycotoxins, such as T-2 toxin, have been shown to induce oxidative stress and contribute to neurotoxicity.

- *Inflammation:* Toxins can trigger an inflammatory response in the brain, leading to the release of pro-inflammatory molecules. Chronic inflammation can disrupt neuronal function and impair cognitive processes. Inflammatory cytokines, such as interleukin-1 beta (IL-1β) and tumor necrosis factor-alpha (TNF-α), have been implicated in toxin-induced cognitive impairment.

- *Disruption of neuronal structure and function:* Toxins can alter the structure and function of neurons, leading to cognitive impairment. For example, lead exposure has been shown to cause morphological changes in neurons and reduce brain weight, cerebellum size, and thickness of the cerebral cortex and hippocampus. These structural changes can impact neuronal connectivity and synaptic function, affecting learning and memory processes.

Toxins can impair memory and cognition through mechanisms such as impaired synaptic function, neurotoxicity, chemical interference with memory processes, oxidative stress, inflammation, and structural changes in the brain. Understanding these specific mechanisms is crucial for assessing and addressing memory problems resulting from toxin exposure.

Addressing Toxin Exposure

In the intricate dance of contemporary living, where toxins lurk in myriad forms, the symphony of cognitive health faces a unique set of challenges. Amid the disharmony of environmental pollutants and dietary pitfalls, the need for strategic approaches to safeguard memory and cognition becomes paramount.

Cognitive impairments, especially those entwined with learning and memory processes, have been identified as potential consequences of toxin exposure. Let's spotlight actionable strategies that empower individuals to navigate this toxin-infused world.

Healthy Diet

Maintaining a healthy diet is fundamental to minimizing toxin exposure and supporting cognitive health. Emphasizing a diverse array of fruits, vegetables, and whole grains ensures a rich supply of antioxidants, vitamins, and minerals—essential components for the body's natural detoxification processes. Opting for organic produce further reduces the risk of exposure to harmful pesticides and herbicides, fostering a nutritionally robust foundation for cognitive well-being.

Adequate Hydration

Proper hydration is a cornerstone of toxin elimination from the body. By ensuring sufficient water intake, individuals support the kidneys in flushing out toxins through urine, promoting optimal bodily functions, including those vital to cognitive processes. Adequate hydration acts as a conduit for the seamless removal of waste products, contributing to an environment conducive to cognitive health.

Mindful Eating Habits

Mindful eating habits play a pivotal role in minimizing toxin exposure from food sources. Conscious choices in selecting and preparing food can mitigate the risk of contamination by heavy metals, pesticides, or pollutants. Practicing awareness around food sources and employing proper handling and cooking methods fosters a safer and healthier culinary approach, reducing the potential impact of toxins on cognitive function.

Limiting Processed Foods

Reducing the consumption of processed foods is a strategic measure in curbing toxin exposure. Processed foods often contain additives, preservatives, and artificial ingredients that may contribute to the body's toxic burden. Opting for whole, minimally processed foods aligns with a holistic approach to nutrition, lowering the likelihood of exposure to harmful substances that could compromise cognitive health.

Environmental Awareness

Maintaining environmental awareness is indispensable for minimizing toxin exposure beyond dietary considerations. Being mindful of environmental factors, such as air pollution and household cleaners, empowers individuals to make informed choices. Selecting eco-friendly products and ensuring proper ventilation in living spaces are actionable steps toward reducing indoor air pollutants and fostering an environment conducive to cognitive well-being.

Regular Exercise

Regular physical activity contributes not only to overall well-being but also to toxin elimination. Engaging in exercise promotes circulation and sweating, facilitating the expulsion of toxins from the body. Beyond its detoxification benefits, regular exercise has been associated with cognitive advantages, underscoring its role in promoting a healthy mind and body.

Effective Stress Management

Stress management is integral to mitigating the impact of toxins on cognitive health. Chronic stress can exacerbate the detrimental effects of toxins, making stress-reducing techniques such as meditation, deep breathing, or yoga essential components of a comprehensive strategy. By fostering resilience against stressors, individuals fortify their cognitive defenses and support long-term brain health.

Quality Sleep

Prioritizing quality sleep is imperative for any strategy focused on minimizing toxin exposure and safeguarding cognitive function. Sleep plays a pivotal role in facilitating essential detoxification and repair processes within the body, allowing it to effectively combat the adverse effects of toxins. Adequate and restorative sleep is indispensable as it forms the cornerstone of maintaining optimal cognitive health. By ensuring that the body receives the necessary rest it needs, individuals can enhance their overall well-being and bolster their cognitive resilience against the detrimental impacts of toxins. Thus, incorporating sufficient sleep into daily routines is essential for promoting long-term cognitive function and overall health.

Limiting Alcohol and Caffeine

Moderating the intake of alcohol and caffeine is a prudent measure to ease the strain on the liver, a central organ in detoxification. Excessive consumption of these substances can contribute to toxin accumulation, potentially impairing cognitive function. Striking a balance through moderation fosters a supportive environment for cognitive health.

Regular Health Check-ups

Scheduled health check-ups serve as proactive measures to identify and address potential toxin exposure or related health issues. Early detection enables timely intervention and prevention,

DAVID L. PRIEDE, PHD

allowing individuals to take preemptive steps toward maintaining optimal cognitive function. Regular check-ups form a critical component of a comprehensive health strategy.

Environmental Consciousness

Supporting environmental conservation initiatives and advocating for reduced industrial pollutants extends the commitment to minimizing toxin exposure beyond individual practices. Contributing to broader efforts in environmental consciousness aligns with a collective responsibility to create a healthier, less toxic environment for all, positively impacting cognitive health on a societal level.

Professional Advice

Seeking guidance from healthcare professionals or environmental specialists provides personalized insights based on individual circumstances. This approach ensures a tailored strategy for reducing toxin exposure, incorporating expert knowledge to address specific concerns and promote cognitive well-being effectively. Professional advice acts as a valuable resource in crafting a comprehensive plan for toxin reduction.

In weaving these practices into daily life, individuals can foster a proactive and holistic approach to reducing toxin exposure, fortifying their cognitive resilience, and promoting long-term brain health. Each element contributes synergistically to create an environment that supports cognitive well-being, emphasizing the interconnectedness of lifestyle choices and their profound impact on cognitive health.

Igniting the Flame for Toxin-Induced Memory Loss Research and Awareness

As evidence linking toxins to memory loss and cognitive decline continues to accumulate, it becomes increasingly crucial to illuminate the critical intersection between environmental health and cognitive well-being. This urgent call to action impels researchers, advocates, and the public to join forces in a collective endeavor.

Together, we must embark on a shared mission: to delve deeper into the complex mechanisms underlying toxin-induced memory impairments and to elevate awareness initiatives to unprecedented levels of impact.

In recognizing the profound implications of environmental toxins on cognitive function, we acknowledge the pressing need for comprehensive research efforts aimed at unraveling the intricacies of this relationship. By fostering collaboration across disciplines and harnessing cutting-edge technologies, we can gain invaluable insights into the pathways through which toxins exert their deleterious effects on memory and cognition.

Moreover, this call to action extends beyond the realms of academia and scientific inquiry. It implores policymakers, healthcare professionals, and community leaders to prioritize initiatives aimed at mitigating toxin exposure and promoting cognitive resilience. Through advocacy campaigns, educational outreach, and policy reforms, we can empower individuals with the knowledge and resources needed to safeguard their cognitive health in the face of environmental challenges.

Ultimately, by uniting in our commitment to addressing the nexus of toxins and cognitive decline, we have the opportunity to effectuate meaningful change on a global scale. Together, we can cultivate a future where every individual has the opportunity to thrive cognitively, unencumbered by the burdens of environmental toxins.

Fueling Research Endeavors

Embarking on a journey of comprehensive exploration, we urge the allocation of resources towards extensive research endeavors that delve into the intricate mechanisms by which toxins impact memory and cognitive function.

It is important to prioritize interdisciplinary studies that bridge gaps between neurotoxicology, environmental science, and cognitive neuroscience, fostering a holistic comprehension of the issue. By doing so, we lay the foundation for groundbreaking insights that can inform targeted interventions and preventive strategies.

Empowering Public Awareness Campaigns

Launching robust public awareness campaigns stands as a cornerstone of this call to action. These initiatives are designed to disseminate accessible information about the potential dangers of toxin exposure on memory.

Utilizing diverse platforms, from social media to community events, we aim to reach a broad audience and foster informed decision-making regarding lifestyle choices that impact cognitive health. Empowering individuals with knowledge becomes a potent tool for creating a society that prioritizes cognitive well-being.

Collaborative Efforts for Policy Advocacy

To effect lasting change, we must engage with policymakers to advocate for regulations and policies that minimize toxin exposure in various spheres of life, from industrial practices to consumer products.

By mobilizing communities to actively participate in discussions and initiatives aimed at creating toxin-reduced environments, we can influence systemic change. This collaborative effort for policy advocacy is pivotal in creating a supportive framework that aligns with cognitive health objectives.

Education Initiatives Across Generations

Integration of educational modules on toxin-induced memory loss into school curricula becomes a crucial step in this call to action. Ensuring that the younger generation is equipped with the knowledge to make informed choices regarding their cognitive health is imperative.

Beyond classrooms, we aim to establish community workshops and seminars that empower individuals of all ages with practical strategies for reducing toxin exposure in their daily lives, fostering a culture of cognitive health awareness.

Encouraging Corporate Responsibility

Engaging with businesses and industries is essential in encouraging sustainable and eco-friendly practices, thereby reducing the release of toxins into the environment. Recognizing and celebrating corporations that prioritize environmental consciousness sets examples for responsible practices that benefit both the workforce and the wider community. This call-to-action urges businesses to view their operations through a cognitive health lens, acknowledging the impact of their choices on the well-being of individuals.

Creating Support Networks

Establishing support networks for individuals experiencing memory loss or cognitive decline linked to toxin exposure is a compassionate dimension of our call to action. These networks provide resources, counseling, and a sense of community to those navigating cognitive health challenges. By fostering collaboration between healthcare professionals, environmental organizations, and community groups, we create comprehensive support systems that address both the physical and emotional aspects of cognitive well-being.

Fostering Global Collaborations

Facilitating international collaborations becomes a cornerstone of this call to action, recognizing that the challenges posed by toxin-induced memory loss are global in scope. By encouraging the exchange of research findings, best practices, and successful strategies in addressing toxin-induced memory loss, we foster a global movement dedicated to cognitive health. This collaborative effort transcends borders, creating a shared commitment to understanding and mitigating the impact of toxins on cognitive well-being.

In heeding this call to action, let us recognize the urgency of the situation and our collective power to effect change. By unifying our efforts in research, awareness, and advocacy, we pave the way for a future where toxin-induced memory loss is not only understood but actively mitigated through informed choices, robust policies, and a shared commitment to cognitive well-being.

Reflections on The Role of Toxins in Memory Loss

The intertwining of toxins and memory loss unravels a compelling narrative of how environmental factors can impact our cognitive well-being. Toxins, whether in the air we breathe, the food we consume, or the substances we encounter, can infiltrate the delicate mechanisms of our brain, leaving a lasting imprint on memory.

The intricate dance between toxins and the brain's intricate circuitry reveals the vulnerability of our memory processes to environmental influences. The cumulative impact of chronic toxin exposure may not only affect immediate memory but also contribute to long-term cognitive decline. Recognizing the role of toxins in memory loss emphasizes the importance of environmental stewardship and adopting lifestyle practices that minimize exposure.

Amidst the cautionary tale of environmental toxins and memory, a narrative of empowerment unfolds. Understanding the impact on memory empowers us to make informed choices, advocating for cleaner environments and habits fostering cognitive resilience. This toxin-memory journey is a call to action, urging protection not only for the air we breathe and the food we consume but also for the vitality of our cognitive landscapes.

The impact demands immediate attention, igniting heightened public awareness. Stealthy intruders like heavy metals mingle with our air, water, and food, disrupting the delicate balance and orchestrating memory processes. Neurotoxicity, oxidative stress, and inflammation further complicate this dance. To combat this menace, we marshal resources for vital research funding and longitudinal studies, unraveling the long-term consequences. Advancing understanding, we develop diagnostic tools and biomarkers to unmask early signs of memory impairments.

Knowledge alone isn't sufficient; we arm the public with education and awareness, empowering them to make informed choices against toxic assault. Raising our voices, we implore policymakers to enact stricter regulations, ensuring cleaner air, purer water, and a sustainable future. In a symphony of collaboration, we unravel the enigma, fortify cognitive fortresses, and safeguard memories. Let's rise to the challenge, emboldened by urgency, paving the way for a world where memories flourish, unburdened by toxic shadows.

CHAPTER 18

The Positive Effects of Music and Memory

Music isn't just a sound; it's a powerful catalyst for memory. Music, especially tied to past experiences, can uniquely trigger vivid memories and emotions. Engaging with music stimulates different brain regions, creating neural connections that enhance cognitive function and memory retention. This profound interplay offers therapeutic benefits, making each note a poignant brushstroke on the canvas of our recollections.

Music is more than just a source of entertainment or a cultural hallmark; it is a universal language that transcends borders and profoundly impacts the human psyche. One of the most intriguing aspects of music is its ability to interact with and enhance our memory. Whether it's recalling the lyrics of a childhood song or experiencing a rush of emotions linked to a specific melody, the interplay between music and memory is both fascinating and beneficial. This chapter delves into the science and the art behind this harmonious relationship, exploring how music can be a powerful tool in memory retention, emotional well-being, and even medical treatment.

Emotional Recall

For individuals who suffer from memory-related illnesses such as Alzheimer's disease, music's emotional resonance can be a key to unlocking suppressed memories and feelings. While spoken language and other types of communication may fail, the impact of a familiar tune can awaken a strong emotional connection, sometimes leading to improved awareness and even cognitive function, however temporarily.

This implies that music can serve as a critical bridge between the patient and their forgotten past, offering emotional comfort and improving the quality of life.

- ***Improved Focus and Concentration:*** Numerous studies have shown that certain types of background music, particularly those without lyrics, can enhance one's ability

166

to concentrate on tasks. This effect isn't limited to studying or academic performance but extends to a range of activities requiring focus, from coding to artistic endeavors. The underlying mechanism here could be related to music's ability to modulate arousal and mood, which in turn can optimize cognitive function.

- *Motor Skill Enhancement:* For athletes, dancers, and musicians, music serves as more than just an auditory pleasure; it acts as a guide or metronome that facilitates the timing, coordination, and execution of complex motor skills. The rhythm serves as a roadmap for movement, allowing individuals to perform intricate tasks more precisely. This highlights music's critical role in training and skill acquisition in various domains.

- *Stress Reduction:* Scientific research has consistently demonstrated that certain genres of music can reduce stress by lowering cortisol levels in the body. A stressed brain is generally poor at memory retention and logical reasoning. By offering a natural way to lower stress, music contributes to a state of mind that is more conducive to cognitive functioning and overall mental well-being.

- *Facilitates Learning:* Particularly in early education, academic information set to a tune can be easier to absorb and remember. This is evident in the countless educational jingles designed to teach children everything from the alphabet to historical events. Beyond mere rote learning, this aspect of music can make the educational process more engaging and enjoyable, potentially fostering a lifelong love for learning.

- *Mood Regulation:* Music's capacity to rapidly change our mood makes it a powerful tool in cognitive psychology. It can take someone from a state of anxiety to calmness or from distraction to focus, making learning and memory retention easier. This suggests that a personalized "soundtrack" could optimize mental performance, enhancing everything from exam scores to job performance.

- *Enhanced Multi-tasking:* Listening to music while performing various tasks can sometimes improve the ability to manage multiple information streams. This might be due to music's impact on the brain's executive functions, which govern planning, attention, and simultaneous processing of different information channels.

- *Neuroplasticity:* Musical training can induce brain structure and function changes, whether playing an instrument or understanding musical theory. These changes improve cognitive flexibility, enhancing the brain's ability to adapt and grow throughout life, which can have long-term benefits on memory and various cognitive functions.
- *Improved Sleep:* A growing body of evidence suggests that specific types of music, usually slow-tempo and calming, can significantly improve sleep quality. Better sleep directly affects cognitive functions such as memory retention, problem-solving abilities, and focus.
- *Cultural and Social Benefits:* Music is a bonding agent in many social situations, from concerts to religious ceremonies. This collective experience enhances our emotional intelligence and allows for a more nuanced understanding of social cues, a key aspect of social cognition.
- *Therapeutic Uses:* As the benefits of music therapy gain scientific credibility, we see more widespread adoption in healthcare, treating conditions ranging from emotional disorders to cognitive impairments. While it is not a substitute for conventional medical treatments, it is an effective adjunct therapy.
- *Enhanced Creativity*: Music's abstract, non-linear nature seems to encourage creative thinking patterns. The improved cognitive flexibility allows individuals to think "outside the box," making it an asset in problem-solving scenarios.
- *Speech and Language Skills:* Exposure to music at an early age has been linked to more advanced language skills in children. Music helps in the understanding of phonetic nuances and can improve both verbal memory and literacy skills. Since cognition and language skills are tightly interconnected, this can have a positive knock-on effect on other areas of cognitive development.

Each of these points provides a comprehensive look into how music interacts with and augments our cognitive functions. These insights are valuable for individual well-being and have broader implications in educational and healthcare systems.

Reflections on The Positive Effects of Music and Memory

The emotional power of music can ignite vivid memories, transporting us back to specific moments, places, or feelings. Music's impact also extends into the realm of skill and motor memory. Athletes, dancers, and musicians leverage music's rhythmic aspects for better timing, coordination, and execution of complex tasks. Music serves as a roadmap for movement, reinforcing muscle memory and enhancing performance.

Whether you are a student aiming to excel in exams, an athlete striving for perfection, or a medical professional seeking alternative treatments for memory-related conditions, the potential benefits of this relationship are too significant to ignore. From a broader perspective, this harmonious relationship between music and memory enriches our lives. It has the potential to bring breakthroughs in the education and healthcare sectors.

The symbiotic relationship between music and memory opens many possibilities for enhancing quality of life, education, and healthcare. As we explore this intricate relationship, one thing remains clear: music is a natural mnemonic device with the power to shape and illuminate our past, present, and future.

Thus, the next time you find yourself lost in a melody or captivated by a rhythm, remember that you are enjoying a piece of art and engaging in an age-old practice that nurtures your memory and enriches your cognitive landscape.

CHAPTER 19

Neuromodulation and Memory Enhancement

Neuromodulation for memory enhancement is a cutting-edge field that involves fine-tuning neural circuits to optimize memory function. It envisions a future where the delicate orchestration of electrical pulses can amplify memory capabilities, marking a synergy between neuroscience and technology and creating an exciting journey at the forefront of memory enhancement.

In recent years, neuromodulation has emerged as a captivating field of research and clinical application, offering new ways to influence neural activity and, thereby, cognitive functions. The application of neuromodulation for memory enhancement is an area of growing interest, offering potentially groundbreaking advancements in neuroscience and medical therapy. One of the most compelling areas of focus within neuromodulation is its potential for enhancing memory.

Neuromodulation techniques have demonstrated the potential to improve memory recall in research and clinical environments. Alongside its effects on recall, neuromodulation is also being studied for its impact on the consolidation and storage of memories, although this remains an area of ongoing research. Additionally, preliminary investigations suggest that neuromodulation could enhance working memory, the type of memory used for holding and manipulating information over short periods. These advancements indicate that neuromodulation offers promising avenues for enhancing various aspects of memory function.

Transcranial Magnetic Stimulation (TMS)

Transcranial Magnetic Stimulation (TMS) is a non-invasive technique that uses magnetic fields to modulate neural activity in specific regions of the brain. Initially developed for treating psychiatric disorders like depression, TMS has also shown promise in studying and potentially enhancing cognitive functions, including memory. This article explores the relationship between TMS and memory, shedding light on how this groundbreaking technology could reshape our understanding of cognitive neuroscience.

TMS works by applying a magnetic coil to the scalp, which generates a magnetic field that penetrates the skull to stimulate underlying neural tissue. Because it's non-invasive and generally well-tolerated, TMS offers an appealing option for researchers investigating brain functions and clinicians treating various neurological and psychiatric conditions.

Studies have begun to illuminate how TMS can influence memory processes. Researchers often target regions like the prefrontal cortex and the hippocampus, which play key roles in memory formation and retrieval. Several findings suggest that TMS can:

- *Enhance memory recall:* Some studies have shown improved performance on memory tasks following TMS application.
- *Interfere with memory:* Conversely, TMS can also disrupt memory processes, providing insights into the regions of the brain that are imperative for specific memory tasks.
- *Influence memory consolidation:* Early evidence suggests that TMS may affect the process of stabilizing memories after they have been initially acquired.

Given its impact on memory, TMS is also being explored as a potential treatment for disorders characterized by memory deficits, such as Alzheimer's disease. While the research is still in preliminary stages, early trials have shown some promise in slowing memory decline in affected patients.

Transcranial Magnetic Stimulation offers a fascinating and promising avenue for studying and potentially enhancing memory. Its non-invasive nature and the depth of its potential applications—from basic neuroscience research to clinical interventions—make it a subject of ongoing interest for scientists and clinicians alike. However, proceeding cautiously and considering the ethical implications as this technology evolves is essential.

Neurofeedback

A more holistic approach to addressing memory-related challenges involves a cutting-edge technique that facilitates healthier brain activity patterns. This technique utilizes a device known as an electroencephalogram (EEG), which plays a pivotal role in tracking and influencing brain activity to promote better memory function.

The EEG is a non-invasive technology that records electrical activity in the brain through electrodes placed on the scalp. This process allows for real-time monitoring of brainwave patterns and provides valuable insights into how the brain functions.

In memory enhancement, the EEG can be employed as a tool to guide the brain toward adopting healthier activity patterns. Here's how it works:

1. *Brain Activity Assessment:* The EEG is initially used to assess an individual's brain activity. This involves recording baseline brainwave patterns to identify areas of concern or irregularities associated with memory function.
2. *Customized Intervention:* A customized intervention plan is developed based on the assessment. This plan involves using the EEG to provide real-time feedback to the individual. This feedback can take various forms, such as visual or auditory cues.
3. *Neurofeedback Training:* The individual actively participates in neurofeedback training sessions while connected to the EEG. During these sessions, they are guided to perform tasks or engage in mental activities that encourage the brain to adopt more optimal and healthier activity patterns related to memory.
4. *Reinforcement and Adaptation:* The brain adapts and rewires itself as the individual consistently engages in neurofeedback sessions. It learns to operate in a manner conducive to improved memory function.

While memory enhancement is one application, EEG-guided neurofeedback has demonstrated efficacy in addressing various neurological and psychological conditions. It has been used successfully in the rehabilitation of individuals with traumatic brain injuries (TBIs), managing post-traumatic stress disorder (PTSD) symptoms, alleviating symptoms of depression, and even assisting in the management of Parkinson's disease.

The power of EEG-guided neurofeedback lies in its ability to harness the brain's inherent neuroplasticity—the brain's capacity to reorganize and adapt its structure and function. This technique empowers individuals to actively participate in their brain's transformation toward healthier memory-related activity patterns by offering real-time feedback and training.

While it may not be a one-size-fits-all solution, EEG-guided neurofeedback represents a promising avenue for enhancing memory and cognitive function while addressing various neurological and psychological challenges. As our understanding of neuroplasticity and brain health continues to evolve, such innovative approaches hold the potential to unlock new possibilities for memory improvement and overall well-being.

Cranial Electrotherapy Stimulation (CES):

Cranial Electrotherapy Stimulation (CES) has been explored as a potential tool for enhancing cognitive functions, including learning. The technique involves the application of a low-level electrical current to the head, often through electrodes clipped to the earlobes or attached to other parts of the head. The idea is that this electrical stimulation may modulate brain activity, potentially leading to improved cognitive performance.

While CES has not been directly correlated with memory enhancement, it could have indirect effects. For example, alleviating symptoms of stress or anxiety could potentially improve cognitive functions, including memory. High-stress levels are known to adversely affect memory, so a treatment that mitigates stress could conceivably positively impact memory as well.

CES is thought to induce the release of neurotransmitters like serotonin and endorphins. These neurotransmitters are involved in mood regulation and play a role in cognitive functions. Therefore, it is plausible that CES could have some influence on memory, although this has not been extensively studied.

Research on the effectiveness of CES for learning is still in its early stages, and the results are mixed. Some studies suggest that CES may positively impact learning and cognitive functions, possibly by affecting neurotransmitter levels or promoting neural plasticity. However, other studies have not found significant benefits, and there is still much debate in the scientific community about the efficacy of CES for cognitive enhancement.

Transcranial Direct Current Stimulation (tDCS)

Transcranial Direct Current Stimulation (tDCS) is a non-invasive form of brain stimulation that involves the application of a constant, low electrical current to the scalp through electrodes. The technique aims to modulate neuronal activity and has been investigated for various applications, including cognitive enhancement, pain management, and treatment of various neurological and psychiatric disorders. In the context of memory, tDCS is thought to potentially influence cognitive functions by altering neurotransmitter levels or facilitating neural plasticity. Research on its efficacy for enhancing memory has produced mixed results, and the scientific community is still debating its effectiveness. The procedure is generally considered safe but may have minor side effects like skin irritation. It is important to consult a healthcare provider for a personalized treatment plan.

tDCS involves the application of a constant, low electrical current to the scalp via electrodes. The current is thought to modulate neuronal activity, which could impact cognitive functions.

Research on the effects of tDCS on memory has produced mixed results. Some studies suggest that tDCS can enhance memory performance, particularly working and long-term memory. The mechanisms behind these effects are not fully understood but may involve changes in neurotransmitter levels or the facilitation of neural plasticity. However, other studies have not found significant benefits, and there is ongoing debate within the scientific community about the efficacy of tDCS for memory enhancement.

As with CES, tDCS is generally considered to be a safe procedure with minimal side effects, such as skin irritation or mild discomfort. However, consulting a healthcare provider for a proper diagnosis and treatment plan tailored to individual needs is Important.

Deep Brain Stimulation (DBS)

Deep Brain Stimulation (DBS) is a medical procedure involving the surgical implantation of electrodes into specific brain regions. These electrodes are connected to a device called a neurostimulator, which is typically placed under the skin in the chest. The neurostimulator sends electrical impulses to the brain, modulating the activity of targeted neural circuits. DBS is adjustable and reversible, allowing clinicians to fine-tune the stimulation parameters to optimize treatment outcomes.

Originally developed to treat movement disorders like Parkinson's disease, DBS has also been studied for its potential in treating various other conditions, such as epilepsy, obsessive-compulsive disorder, and even depression. It is considered a more invasive form of neuromodulation compared to techniques like

Transcranial Magnetic Stimulation (TMS) because it requires surgical implantation.

Although DBS is primarily known for its applications in treating movement and mood disorders, it has also been the subject of research for its effects on memory. Some studies have indicated that DBS, when targeted at specific regions like the hippocampus or fornix—areas closely linked with memory functions—may benefit memory enhancement or stabilization, especially in neurodegenerative diseases like Alzheimer's. However, these findings are still relatively preliminary and require further validation.

DBS for memory enhancement or restoration poses both opportunities and ethical considerations, particularly regarding its long-term effects and potential use for cognitive enhancement beyond therapeutic needs.

Other Neuromodulation Techniques

In addition to Transcranial Magnetic Stimulation (TMS) and Deep Brain Stimulation (DBS), there are several other neuromodulation techniques used in medical practice and research:

- *Transcutaneous Electrical Nerve Stimulation (TENS):* TENS involves the application of electrical stimulation to peripheral nerves through electrodes placed on the skin. It is commonly used to relieve pain.
- *Spinal Cord Stimulation (SCS):* SCS involves the implantation of electrodes along the spinal cord to alleviate chronic pain by modulating the transmission of pain signals.
- *Vagus Nerve Stimulation (VNS):* VNS involves the implantation of a device that delivers electrical impulses to the vagus nerve, which runs from the brainstem to various organs in the body. It is used to treat epilepsy, depression, and other neurological and psychiatric disorders.
- *Peripheral Nerve Stimulation (PNS):* PNS involves the placement of electrodes directly on peripheral nerves outside of the brain and spinal cord. It is used to treat various chronic pain conditions, including neuropathic pain and complex regional pain syndrome.
- *Motor Cortex Stimulation (MCS):* MCS involves the placement of electrodes directly on the motor cortex of the brain. It is used to treat chronic pain conditions, movement

disorders, and certain neurological conditions like stroke and spinal cord injury.

- **Prefrontal Cortex Stimulation:** This technique involves the stimulation of the prefrontal cortex, a region of the brain associated with executive functions, mood regulation, and decision-making. It is being investigated for its potential in treating depression, anxiety, and other psychiatric disorders.
- **Sacral Nerve Stimulation (SNS):** SNS involves the implantation of electrodes near the sacral nerves in the lower back. It is used to treat urinary and fecal incontinence, as well as pelvic pain syndromes.
- **Cochlear Implants:** While primarily used to restore hearing in individuals with severe-to-profound hearing loss, cochlear implants can also be considered a form of neuromodulation. These devices bypass damaged hair cells in the cochlea and directly stimulate the auditory nerve to provide auditory sensations.
- **Intrathecal Drug Delivery (IDD):** IDD involves the delivery of medication directly into the cerebrospinal fluid surrounding the spinal cord via an implanted pump and catheter system. It is used to manage severe chronic pain and spasticity by delivering medications such as opioids, baclofen, and local anesthetics directly to the spinal cord.

These neuromodulation techniques offer promising therapeutic options for individuals with various neurological and psychiatric conditions, although they also raise ethical considerations regarding safety, efficacy, and access to treatment. Continued research and advancements in neuromodulation hold potential for expanding treatment options and improving outcomes for patients with these disorders.

Neuromodulation Ethical Considerations

The growing interest in neuromodulation techniques like Transcranial Magnetic Stimulation (TMS) and Deep Brain Stimulation (DBS) for various medical and cognitive applications inevitably brings a range of ethical considerations. Below are some of the key ethical issues surrounding the use of neuromodulation:

Informed Consent

One of the foremost concerns is the issue of informed consent, especially when dealing with patients who have cognitive impairments or psychiatric conditions. These patients might not be able to fully understand the risks, benefits, and long-term consequences of undergoing neuromodulation, complicating the ethical landscape.

Long-term Safety

While neuromodulation techniques have been generally considered safe for short-term use, the long-term effects on brain health and function are not yet fully understood. This lack of comprehensive safety data raises ethical questions about the appropriateness of using these techniques for non-essential cognitive enhancement or for treating conditions that have alternative treatments with better-understood safety profiles.

Cognitive and Social Inequality

The potential for neuromodulation to enhance cognitive functions like memory could lead to a future where these technologies are widely used for non-therapeutic cognitive enhancement. This opens the door to cognitive and social inequality concerns, where only those who can afford such enhancements benefit, thereby widening existing societal gaps.

Privacy and Autonomy

Neuromodulation techniques could potentially be misused to alter mental states or even manipulate thoughts and behaviors without consent, leading to concerns about individual autonomy and privacy. This is especially concerning in scenarios where neuromodulation could be used coercively or without full transparency.

Accessibility

As cutting-edge technologies, neuromodulation techniques are often expensive and not universally available, leading to ethical concerns about who gets access to these potentially life-changing treatments. There may be disparities in access based on socioeconomic status, geographic location, or healthcare systems.

Slippery Slope to Unintended Applications

As research advances, there's a potential for neuromodulation to be applied in ways not initially intended or ethically questionable. For example, could these technologies be used for military applications, such as creating soldiers who feel less pain or fear?

While neuromodulation holds significant promise for treating a variety of medical conditions and enhancing human cognition, its ethical implications are complex and multifaceted. As such, regulatory agencies, ethicists, clinicians, and researchers must collaborate closely to navigate these ethical challenges responsibly.

Reflections on Neuromodulation and Memory Enhancement

The field of neuromodulation unfolds as a promising frontier in the ongoing quest for memory enhancement, offering an enthralling journey into the convergence of technology and cognitive prowess. This cutting-edge approach involves the precise modulation of neural circuits to optimize memory functions, ushering in a new era of possibilities in the realm of human cognition.

Imagine a symphony where neuromodulation serves as the conductor, orchestrating the delicate harmonies of our neural networks. Techniques such as transcranial magnetic stimulation (TMS) or deep brain stimulation (DBS) emerge as instruments capable of finely tuning the dynamics of memory formation, consolidation, and retrieval.

What sets neuromodulation apart is its remarkable precision, empowering researchers and clinicians to navigate the neural symphony with unparalleled accuracy. By selectively stimulating or inhibiting specific brain regions, this technique holds the potential to enhance memory in a targeted manner, addressing cognitive challenges at their core.

In the vast landscape of memory research, neuromodulation emerges as a prominent protagonist, shedding light on the brain's remarkable plasticity and its capacity for improvement. It invites us to envision a future where memory enhancement transcends the realm of possibility to become a tangible reality—a future where the symphony of our neural networks can be finely tuned to compose the harmonious melodies of an enriched cognitive experience.

CHAPTER 20

Using Mnemonics for Enhanced Memory

Whether you're a student grappling with academic overload or a professional juggling multiple responsibilities, the magic key may be mnemonics. These memory aids are not merely tricks or shortcuts but tools that transform abstract complexities into vivid, memorable experiences. Welcome to the extraordinary power of the mind, made accessible through mnemonics. Harness these tools to remember better, elevate your understanding, and enrich your daily life.

Memory is one of the most captivating and mysterious aspects of the human experience. It's an essential tool we all depend on for everything from simple tasks like remembering grocery lists and birthdays to more complex cognitive feats like mastering mathematical formulas. Yet, our memory can be inconsistent, often leaving us in the lurch when we need it most. Enter mnemonics, the age-old art of memory enhancement that has been helping people optimize their cognitive functions for centuries.

Derived from the name of Mnemosyne, the Ancient Greek goddess of memory, mnemonics serve as mental aids to help us remember information more effectively. They work by providing a structured framework that organizes data in a way that is easier for the brain to retrieve later.

Imagine turning your brain into a highly organized filing system, where every bit of information has its specific location, easily accessible when needed.

Mnemonics come in various forms: a catchy rhyme, a vivid image, an easily recalled phrase, or a simple acronym. These tools take advantage of our brain's natural ability to recognize patterns and make associations, allowing us to retrieve information more easily. In essence, mnemonics offer a form of cognitive 'scaffolding' that enables us to elevate our memory capabilities.

Integrating mnemonics into your daily life enhances your ability to remember and take a proactive step toward harnessing your brain's full potential.

Mnemonic Techniques

Mnemonic techniques are structured methods that leverage our brain's natural propensity for pattern recognition and association. Whether you're a student, a professional, or someone interested in cognitive improvement, understanding these techniques can offer practical tools for better memory retention and retrieval.

Let's explore various types of mnemonic techniques, each with its unique approach and application, to help you unlock the full potential of your memory.

Acronyms and Acrostics

An acronym is a specific type of mnemonic where the first letter of each word in a list or phrase is used to form a new word that is easier to remember. For instance, the acronym "PEMDAS" is commonly used in mathematics to remember the order of operations: Parentheses, Exponents, Multiplication and Division, and Addition and Subtraction. The acronym becomes a simple, easy-to-remember word that stands for a more complex set of information. It's like a memory shortcut, taking you directly to the details you need to recall.

Acrostics, like acronyms, have a slight twist. Instead of forming a new word, the first letters of each item in the list are used to create a memorable sentence or phrase. For example, "My Very Educated Mother Just Served Us Noodles" is an acrostic that helps people remember the order of planets in our solar system: Mercury, Venus, Earth, Mars, Jupiter, Saturn, Uranus, and Neptune. Acrostics offer a narrative framework for remembering lists, transforming them into something more relatable and easier to visualize. This makes the content easier to retrieve from memory later.

Both acronyms and acrostics are valuable tools for a wide range of applications. Students might use them to remember historical dates, elements on the periodic table, or the stages of mitosis. Professionals might use acronyms to recall technical specifications or steps in a project management process. Regardless of the field, these techniques make challenging lists or sequences more manageable and easier to remember.

Rhymes, Songs, and Jingles

Rhymes and songs as mnemonic devices exploit the powerful link between music and memory, turning remembering into an engaging and enjoyable activity. Our brains are naturally wired to recognize patterns and rhythms, so musical mnemonics can make information stick in our minds for extended periods. For example, the "Alphabet Song" utilizes a catchy melody to teach children the sequence of the alphabet, transforming a potentially challenging learning experience into a playful and memorable one.

The effectiveness of this method is not limited to educational settings. In the commercial world, jingles have proven incredibly impactful in creating brand recognition. Advertisers ensure their message is heard and remembered by adding product names, slogans, or services to a melody. This is why you might find yourself involuntarily recalling a jingle for a product you haven't thought about in years; the auditory and musical elements make it sticky in your memory.

Music and rhymes work by tying the information to be remembered to a specific auditory pattern or tune. This stimulates multiple brain areas responsible for auditory processing, language comprehension, and emotional response. Because of this multi-faceted engagement, rhymes and songs serve as highly effective mnemonic devices, offering versatile applications. Whether you are a student trying to master a complex scientific formula, a professional seeking to remember industry-specific terminology, or simply someone aiming to make daily life a little easier, rhymes and songs can be your allies in achieving better memory retention.

Method of Loci (Memory Palace)

The Method of Loci, commonly called the Memory Palace technique, is a time-honored mnemonic strategy that offers a compelling way to boost memory. Originating from the ancient Greeks and Romans, this technique turns remembering into a vivid, spatial journey. You create a mental map that guides you through memory recall by tying information to specific geographical or architectural landmarks in a familiar setting.

The first step in utilizing the Method of Loci is to select a space you know exceptionally well—be it your home, a regular walking route, or even a favorite vacation spot. This space will serve as the "palace" in your Memory Palace technique. Next, identify specific landmarks within this space, such as home furniture or park trees. These landmarks will serve as pegs on which you "hang" the information you wish to remember.

For example, suppose you are trying to remember a grocery list. In that case, you might start at the front door of your home as the first landmark and associate it with the first item on your list, like milk. Then, as you mentally move through your home—perhaps to the living room—you associate the second landmark, like the couch, with the second item on your list, such as bread. The key is to make the association as vivid and detailed as possible, perhaps adding an emotional or humorous element to make the memory more resilient.

When recalling the list or sequence, you stroll through your designated "palace," allowing each landmark to trigger the memory of its associated item. This method is incredibly effective and is often used by memory athletes in competitions to remember vast amounts of data with remarkable accuracy.

The beauty of the Method of Loci lies in its adaptability and scalability. You can use it for short lists or scale it up for complex information like historical timelines or medical procedures. Its utility spans numerous disciplines, from academic and professional settings to daily life tasks. By exploiting the brain's natural aptitude for spatial memory, the Method of Loci elevates your memory ability, making it a powerful tool in your cognitive arsenal.

Chunking and Grouping

Chunking is a mnemonic technique that capitalizes on the brain's natural propensity for organization. By breaking down extensive strings of information into smaller, more manageable "chunks," the cognitive load on your memory is reduced, making it easier to absorb and recall information. This technique is rooted in the psychological theory that our working memory can only hold a limited amount of information simultaneously. Therefore, organizing this data into smaller units can enhance our ability to remember it.

Take phone numbers, for example. Instead of trying to remember a continuous string of ten digits, we often break them down into smaller units: the area code, the first three numbers, and the last four numbers. This segmented approach makes the number significantly easier to remember and retrieve when needed.

Another variant of chunking is known as grouping. In this approach, you arrange similar or related items into categories to facilitate memory recall. For example, suppose your grocery list contains various fruits and vegetables along with other things. In that case, you might group all the fruits and all the vegetables. By categorizing the items, you create smaller, meaningful clusters of information that can be recalled more effortlessly.

Chunking and grouping are not just limited to numbers or lists; they can also be applied to more complex sets of information. When studying for exams, students often use these techniques to break down intricate concepts or large chapters into digestible sections. Professionals might use chunking in project management to divide a large project into smaller, more manageable tasks.

In essence, chunking and grouping are adaptable strategies that cater to the limitations of our working memory. By reorganizing the information landscape into smaller units or categories, these techniques make it easier to commit information to long-term memory and retrieve it later. They can be a boon for anyone looking to enhance their memory capabilities for academic purposes, professional development, or daily life activities.

Visual Imagery and Storytelling

Visual mnemonics harness the power of vivid, mental imagery to enhance memory retention and recall. This technique works exceptionally well because the brain can quickly process and remember images rather than abstract concepts or words. In visual mnemonics, the aim is often to create the most outrageous, bizarre, or emotionally charged images. The more distinctive the image, the more likely it will stick in your memory. For example, suppose you're trying to remember the order of planets in the solar system. In that case, you might imagine a gigantic Mercury thermometer bursting in the sun, followed by a Venus flytrap eating Earth. The wilder the image, the more memorable it becomes.

Building on the concept of visual mnemonics is the method of storytelling. Instead of creating isolated images for individual pieces of information, you weave those images or ideas into a cohesive, engaging narrative. This narrative context provides additional cues that help retrieve the information. For example, if you're studying for a history exam, instead of simply remembering dates and names, you could create a storyline involving key figures participating in dramatic events, like a dialogue between philosophers or a battle scene involving historical generals.

Storytelling can be particularly potent when remembering information in a specific order. Just as in a well-plotted story, each piece of information (or character, event, etc.) leads logically or dramatically to the next, making the sequence easier to remember. You're essentially constructing a mental movie or a play where the information you need to recall plays a pivotal role.

Both visual mnemonics and storytelling capitalize on the human brain's affinity for images and stories. These techniques make learning more enjoyable and significantly boost memory retention and recall. Whether you're a student looking to master complicated subjects or a professional needing to remember a series of tasks or objectives, these techniques offer a creative and effective way to optimize your memory.

Peg Method

The Peg Method is a creative way to remember a list of items by linking them to a sequence you already know, like numbers or the alphabet. The 'peg' is a mental hook where you can 'hang' the information you need to recall. You would pair each item on your list with a number to get started. For example, if you need to remember to buy milk, bread, and eggs, you'd associate milk with the number one, bread with the number two, and eggs with the number three.

Here's where it gets fun: to make the memory stick, you'd visualize an exaggerated or silly scenario combining the number and the item. Imagine a giant 'one' pouring milk into a huge cereal bowl or a 'two' made of bread. These mental images act as cues that trigger your memory when remembering the items on your list. The more unique and absurd the imagery, the easier it is to recall the list later.

The Peg Method is beneficial for remembering ordered lists, like directions or steps in a process, as the sequence of 'pegs' can help you recognize the correct order of items. This makes the method highly versatile and applicable for everything from grocery shopping to presentation preparation.

Keyword Method

The Keyword Method is an ingenious technique geared toward helping you remember new vocabulary, especially when learning a foreign language or grappling with specialized terminology. The first step involves identifying a 'keyword,' which is a word that sounds similar to the new word you're trying to remember and is in a language you already know. The power of the Keyword Method lies in its next step: creating a vivid mental image that links the meaning of the unfamiliar word to this keyword. For instance, if you're learning the Spanish word "gato," which means 'cat,' you might link it to the similar-sounding English word 'gate.' You could visualize a quirky scenario where a cat sits atop a gate or jumps over it. This memorable image acts as a mental anchor, helping you instantly recall the meaning of "gato" whenever you hear it.

The technique goes beyond repetition and memorization by engaging multiple cognitive faculties, including auditory perception, linguistic understanding, and imaginative visualization. This multi-sensory approach enhances retention and makes the learning process more engaging. The Keyword Method is especially useful for students tackling new academic terminology or for language enthusiasts wanting to expand their vocabulary. It offers an efficient and creative way to turn a daunting learning task into a series of memorable mental snapshots.

Concept Mapping and Diagrams

Concept Mapping and Diagrams serve as potent visual tools that cater to those inclined toward visual or spatial learning. These are not your run-of-the-mill notetaking or list-making techniques; they transform nebulous or complicated ideas into a clear and structured visual representation, making the information more accessible and easier to recall.

In a concept map, the spotlight is on a central idea or theme, which radiates to subsidiary topics or related notions. Lines or arrows link these components, and these connections are often annotated to describe the nature of the relationship between the ideas. This creates an interconnected web, allowing for an at-a-glance understanding of how various elements relate. This is highly beneficial for deepening comprehension and facilitating memory retention. It is helpful in educational settings or any scenario where understanding relationships between ideas is key.

Flowcharts are another variant, yet they adopt a more linear, procedural approach. These diagrams are instrumental for delineating sequences, workflows, or multistep processes. Each box in a flowchart represents a specific action or stage, and arrows guide the observer through the sequence of activities. This linear mapping is invaluable in fields requiring an understanding of step-by-step processes, such as programming, engineering, or project management, as it allows easy troubleshooting and process optimization.

Concept Mapping and Flowcharts provide a tangible framework for grappling with abstract ideas or complex systems. They are instrumental in academic settings for understanding theories and models, in business settings for workflow analysis, or even in personal life for decision-making and problem-solving.

Applications Across Fields

Mnemonics are not just limited to classroom learning or personal memory tricks; their applications stretch across many fields. From healthcare and law enforcement to technology and the arts, mnemonics have proven invaluable tools for professionals needing to memorize and recall indispensable information.

This section explores how these versatile memory aids have been adapted to meet the unique demands of various industries, demonstrating that mnemonics are a universal key to unlocking cognitive potential.

Healthcare

In the medical field, mnemonics are quick and efficient ways for healthcare professionals to recall vast amounts of critical information. For example, the acronym "FAST" is used to identify the signs of a stroke: Face drooping, Arm weakness, Speech difficulties, and Time to call emergency services. Mnemonics are also used in medical education to remember complex anatomical terms, steps of surgical procedures, or lists of symptoms associated with specific conditions. This aids in faster and more accurate diagnoses and treatment plans.

Law and Law Enforcement

Legal professionals must often keep many statutes, legal definitions, and procedures in mind. Mnemonics are handy for remembering intricate legal codes or steps in judicial processes. For law enforcement officers, mnemonics like "Miranda" serve as mental prompts to ensure that they adhere to protocol when arresting and informing individuals of their rights, reducing the chance of procedural errors that could compromise cases.

Engineering

Engineers work with complex systems and formulas. A classic example of mnemonics in electrical engineering is "ELI the ICE man," which aids in remembering the phase relationships between voltage and current in inductive and capacitive circuits. Mnemonics help engineers quickly recall these formulas during problem-solving, making their workflow more efficient.

Aviation

Pilots deal with various control systems and emergency protocols that require swift action and accurate memory. Mnemonics like "CIGAR" help them run through essential pretakeoff checks, covering Controls, Instruments, Gas, Airframe, and Run-up. Pilots can ensure they follow the safest operating procedures by memorizing these sequences through mnemonics.

Music

Musicians use mnemonics to remember sequences in scales, finger placements, or notes on a musical staff. For example, "Every Good Boy Deserves Fudge" corresponds to the lines of the treble clef (E, G, B, D, F). Such mnemonics facilitate quicker learning and greater ease in performing, allowing musicians to focus more on artistic expression rather than note recall.

Language Learning

When learning a new language, mnemonics are invaluable for vocabulary retention. Students often create mnemonics to link a foreign word's phonetic sound or meaning to a familiar word or image. This aids in quicker recall during conversations or exams, accelerating language learning.

Psychology

Therapists often use mnemonics to teach their patients coping strategies or cognitive behavioral techniques. For example, the acronym "STOP" can be used to remember the steps of a stress-reduction technique: Stop, take a breath, Observe, and Proceed. Mnemonics are also used in psychological research to explore memory processes.

Education

Educators deploy mnemonics to make learning more engaging and efficient. Teachers might use a rhyme or acronym to help students remember historical dates, mathematical formulas, or the periodic table. These mnemonic devices make the information more accessible to recall and the learning experience more enjoyable.

Everyday Life

In our day-to-day activities, mnemonics offer practical utility. Whether it's remembering a grocery list, directions, or simple chores, mnemonics convert everyday tasks into easy-to-recall formats, enhancing our daily productivity and reducing the chances of forgetting essential items or tasks.

By tailoring mnemonics to each field's specific needs and challenges, professionals and individuals can optimize their memory performance and improve overall efficiency.

Reflections on Using Mnemonics for Enhanced Memory

Let's face it: in a modern world teeming with data, alerts, and endless to-dos, who hasn't experienced the exasperation of forgetting something important? Whether it's a new colleague's name, an essential appointment, or an answer on a test, these lapses can be frustrating and consequential. Mnemonics are not just tricks but systematic techniques that can impact how you remember things. Mnemonics can be likened to an excellent personal assistant who knows how to organize information in a way you can access it.

Mnemonics serve as invaluable memory aids across different facets of life. For students overwhelmed with academic information, they act as organizational tools that make study sessions more efficient and tests more manageable. Professionals also benefit from mnemonics, using them to keep track of indispensable details like client information and deadlines, thus avoiding awkward lapses in memory during important moments. In essence, mnemonics offer a targeted and effective way to improve memory, whether studying for exams or managing a busy work schedule.

But mnemonics aren't only for the high-stakes parts of life. They can be handy for everyday tasks, too. Do you need to remember a shopping list or the sequence of a yoga routine? Mnemonics are versatile enough to be tailored to your daily needs, transforming ordinary tasks into memorable moments.

So, the next time you find yourself wrestling with your memory, know you're not helpless. Reach into your mental toolkit and pull-out mnemonics to give you the needed edge. By integrating these helpful techniques into your cognitive routine, you're not just remembering better—you're also taking a proactive step toward enriching your life and unlocking your brain's full potential.

CHAPTER 21

The Illusion of Memory: Unveiling Imperfections

Forgetting serves as a natural filter for information. Still, it can become problematic when it disrupts our daily lives or impedes our long-term objectives. Whether forgetting someone's name, losing track of keys, or failing to remember important details, these memory slips can act as instructive moments. These lapses shed light on why we forget, aiding in developing memory-boosting strategies and turning setbacks into opportunities for mental growth.

Have you ever struggled to recall a word while chatting with a friend? Or perhaps you've lost your train of thought amidst a noisy environment? While such memory lapses can be frustrating, they're often a normal part of human cognition. Memory isn't infallible; sometimes, specific details slip through the cracks. However, by recognizing these imperfections, we can adopt strategies to improve them.

Memory is a dynamic function, with its reliability and accuracy influenced by various factors. Some of these lapses become more prominent as we grow older. A typical memory challenge is forgetting, which entails an inability to access previously stored data.

Reasons for forgetting include interference, decay, and retrieval failure. Interference emerges when new knowledge hampers the recall of older information. Decay represents the natural fading of memories over time. Retrieval failure arises when cues to prompt a memory are absent or ineffective.

Emotions play a pivotal role in how memories form and are retrieved. Powerful emotional experiences tend to solidify memories, making them easier to recall and more vivid. However, emotion can also warp our recollections, introducing inaccuracies or biases. Research suggests that negatively perceived memories often stand out more distinctly over extended periods than positive ones.

Various elements like age, sleep quality, diet, physical activity, and social interaction can also influence memory efficiency. For instance, aging might impact specific memory functions, particularly those involving working memory. Though we can't alter certain factors like aging, we can influence others. Proper sleep, key for memory consolidation, can boost our ability to form and access memories. The upcoming section will describe typical memory lapses.

The Top Flaws of Memory

When it comes to our memory abilities, we can store many different types. You may be able to recall what your favorite sweatshirt feels like or the details from a field day you had years ago in elementary school. Whether you have powerful memory abilities or are concerned your memory might be slipping, it is essential to recognize that nearly all of us have flawed memories.

Memory imperfections are an inherent part of the human experience, reminding us that our memory system is far from infallible. These imperfections occur due to various factors and can manifest differently, often leading to amusing and frustrating situations. Here are some insights into the fascinating world of memory imperfections:

Tip-of-the-Tongue Phenomenon

The Tip-of-the-Tongue (TOT) Phenomenon is a familiar memory experience in which a person knows they possess a particular piece of information but finds it momentarily elusive, just "on the tip of the tongue." It's like being teased by your own memory, highlighting the intricacies of memory retrieval.

During these moments, a person feels strongly connected to the elusive information. For instance, they might be sure of certain aspects of the word they're trying to remember—perhaps its first letter or its general meaning—but the exact word remains just out of grasp.

Imagine trying to remember the name of an actor known for action films. You might know their name starts with "A" and can even recall specific roles or catchphrases associated with them, yet their full name frustratingly evades you.

Psychologists and cognitive scientists find the TOT Phenomenon intriguing as it provides a glimpse into the complexities of how memories are stored and retrieved. It unveils layers within our memory system and demonstrates how, with patience or external prompts, the memory retrieval process can eventually unearth the elusive piece of information.

Misplaced Memories

In misplaced memories, you vividly recall events or details, only to realize later that these memories aren't as accurate as you initially thought. It's as if these memories have been "misplaced" regarding their fidelity to the actual events. This happens because memory is often reconstructive. When you reminisce about past experiences, your brain tends to assemble information from various sources. Unfortunately, this process can introduce errors or inaccuracies.

Consider a scenario where you recall a childhood birthday party with intricate specifics like a famous cartoon character appearing or an unusually lavish number of presents. However, as you delve deeper, perhaps by looking at old photographs or chatting with family members, you discover that there was no famous character, and the number of gifts was far fewer than you remembered. In this instance, your memory of the event has been misplaced, with elements of fiction blended into the experience.

Misplaced memories are a common type of memory imperfection and offer a clear reminder of the fallibility of our memory system. They underscore how our memories can evolve and change over time, sometimes leading us to believe in events or details that never actually transpired.

False Memories

False memories are intriguing and sometimes unsettling phenomena that can profoundly affect an individual's recollection of events. Imagine this scenario: You're in therapy, discussing your past with a therapist who asks probing questions about your childhood. As you delve into your memories, you suddenly recall a traumatic event from your early years, which you had completely forgotten until now. The memory feels vivid and real, but could it be false?

False memories are fictitious or fabricated recollections of events, situations, or details that feel as genuine and vivid as authentic memories. These can either be entirely fabricated, meaning they never happened, or they can involve distortions of actual events, making them a perplexing aspect of human memory.

False memories can occur for various reasons, including:

- *Suggestive Questioning:* One way that false memories can emerge is through suggestive questioning. Suppose your therapist inadvertently plants inaccurate information by asking leading or suggestive questions during your session.

These questions may lead you to believe in the existence of events that never occurred, shaping your recollections.

- **_Exposure to Misleading Information:_** Another avenue to false memories is exposure to misleading information. Imagine hearing someone else's account of an event that contains inaccuracies. Over time, those inaccuracies can creep into your memory, blurring the line between reality and fiction.

- **_Imagination Inflation:_** Engaging in vivid imagination or visualization can also contribute to false memories. As you repeatedly imagine scenarios related to an event, these imagined experiences can seamlessly integrate into your memory as actual occurrences.

- **_Social Pressure:_** Social pressure and group dynamics play a role, too. Picture a situation where you and your friends remember an event differently. There's a tendency to conform to the group's version of the story, even if it contradicts your initial recollections.

- **_Source Confusion:_** Source confusion, or source amnesia, can further fuel false memories. This happens when you remember information but forget where or how you obtained it. Consequently, you may attribute that information to a different source, leading to distorted memories.

One of the most notable instances of false memories revolves around cases where individuals, during therapy, believe they've recovered previously repressed memories, especially those concerning childhood abuse. Such instances have raised significant controversies.

Some argue that suggestive therapeutic techniques might inadvertently plant these memories, making them seem real to the patient even when they might not have happened.

The existence and implications of false memories touch many facets of human existence. Realizing that our memories can be flawed or even completely fabricated underscores the importance of being discerning and cautious, especially in situations with severe consequences, such as legal cases.

Researchers persist in their investigations into the phenomenon of false memories, striving to comprehend the mechanisms behind them and devising ways to mitigate their potential adverse effects on individuals and society.

Selective Memory

Selective memory is a cognitive phenomenon where people remember specific events, facts, or details while conveniently forgetting or ignoring others. This type of memory bias is often influenced by personal beliefs, biases, emotional attachments, or external influences, and it can significantly impact decision-making and perceptions of reality. Here are some examples to illustrate selective memory:

Confirmation Bias

Confirmation bias is a selective memory where people tend to remember and emphasize information confirming their beliefs or opinions while downplaying or disregarding contradictory information. For instance, in a political context, a person might readily remember and share news articles that support their political views but forget or dismiss articles that challenge them.

Relationships and Personal History

People may selectively remember positive memories and experiences with a partner, friend, or family member in personal relationships while minimizing or forgetting negative interactions. This selective recall can influence how they perceive the overall quality of the relationship.

Emotional Attachments

People often remember events or details associated with strong emotions more vividly than neutral experiences. For example, someone might recognize the specific details of a romantic proposal but forget the mundane aspects of their daily routine during that time.

Forgotten Promises or Obligations

Selective memory can extend to forgetting promises or obligations that people find inconvenient or burdensome. For instance, someone might need to remember a commitment to help a friend move because they would rather not participate in the task.

Biased Interpretation of Past Actions

In conflicts or disagreements, individuals may selectively remember their actions and statements in a more favorable light while recalling the actions and words of others negatively or critically. This bias can reinforce their perspective in a dispute.

Historical Events

In addition to individual perspectives shaping the remembrance of historical events, societal narratives, and cultural influences also play significant roles in shaping collective memory. The portrayal of historical events in media, education systems, and public discourse can further mold and perpetuate certain interpretations while marginalizing others.

This phenomenon highlights the complex interplay between personal memory biases and broader sociocultural factors in shaping our understanding of the past. Therefore, fostering an awareness of these dynamics and actively engaging in diverse perspectives and sources of information is crucial for cultivating a more nuanced and inclusive understanding of history.

Memory Decay

Memory decay is the natural cognitive phenomenon where memories weaken or fade over time. This weakening can affect the recall of specific details, events, or previously encoded information. As time progresses, memories become less vivid, leading to challenges in recalling names, dates, or past events.

However, not all memories fade at the same pace; their decay rate varies based on the strength of the original memory and its rehearsal frequency.

Despite this natural process, not all memories are destined to fade. Strategies like regular review, rehearsal, and mnemonic techniques can combat the effects of memory decay, enhancing retention. Some memories, especially those with deep emotional significance or solid encoding, resist decay better than others. Recognizing how memory decay works is Important for those aiming to bolster their memory performance and retain essential details.

Source Amnesia

Source amnesia, or source misattribution, refers to remembering specific information but forgetting or incorrectly identifying its origin. This means individuals can recall certain facts but are uncertain about where or how they acquired them. Such memory lapses can lead to misplaced trust in information, assuming it to be accurate, original, or reliable when it might not be.

For instance, a person might believe a rumor without remembering where they heard it. In academic contexts, students might remember a fact but forget which book or lecture it came

194

from. In legal scenarios, a witness's testimony might be influenced by source amnesia, causing them to associate details with the wrong event or timeframe.

The phenomenon underscores the intricacies of how memories are formed and retrieved. It emphasizes the need to approach information critically and be constantly aware of its source. To counteract source amnesia, it's beneficial to develop habits like noting down where you obtain specific pieces of information, which can serve as a reliable reference later.

Cryptomnesia

Cryptomnesia is when an individual mistakenly believes they've conceived a fresh, original idea. Still, they're recalling a previously encountered memory or source. It's like the brain's version of "déjà vu" for creativity. Often emerging during creative endeavors, such as writing or composing music, a person, under the influence of cryptomnesia, inadvertently reproduces a thought or concept they've been exposed to in the past, genuinely believing it's their original work.

In the realm of creativity, this can sometimes lead to unintentional imitation or even accusations of plagiarism when the true origin of the idea is recognized. This memory lapse doesn't arise from deliberate intent to copy but rather from the complex interactions of memory, creativity, and the subconscious.

A memory may reside in our brain, lurking beneath conscious awareness. During moments of creation, it can resurface, masquerading as a fresh insight.

For those immersed in creative fields, being vigilant about their inspirations can help to sidestep cryptomnesia. This might involve maintaining meticulous notes on references, conducting exhaustive checks on their work, and being consciously present during the creative process, ever aware of the fine line between inspiration and replication.

Prospective Memory Failures

Prospective memory failures refer to instances when people fail to remember to perform a planned action or task in the future, at a specified time, or in a particular context. Prospective memory involves remembering to do something in the future, and it can be classified into two main categories: event-based prospective memory and time-based prospective memory.

1. ***Event-based Prospective Memory:*** This involves remembering to act in response to a specific event or cue.

195

For example, remembering to buy groceries when passing by a grocery store or to send a birthday card when receiving a reminder.

2. **Time-based Prospective Memory:** This entails remembering to perform an action at a specific time or after a certain amount of time has passed. Examples include taking medication at a prescribed time or attending a meeting at a scheduled hour.

Prospective memory failures can happen due to factors such as distraction, information overload, emotional stress, or even age-related cognitive decline. These lapses can disrupt planned activities and tasks, making understanding their underlying causes for effective management and improvement critical.

Distractions

External factors like noise, visual stimuli, or the presence of other tasks can significantly impact prospective memory. The likelihood of forgetting increases when attention is drawn away from the intended future task. This can happen when an individual is multitasking or preoccupied with other matters, making it harder to recall and execute the planned action.

Memory Retrieval Difficulties

Sometimes, despite having a mental note of the intended task, people may struggle to bring it to conscious awareness when needed. This can be due to various reasons, such as memory interference from other similar tasks or a lack of focus when the action needs to be carried out. Failure to retrieve the memory at the appropriate time can result in a missed opportunity or a task left undone.

Stress and Cognitive Load

High stress levels or a heavy cognitive load can take a toll on prospective memory. When the mind is preoccupied with pressing concerns, it allocates more resources to managing the immediate situation, often at the expense of future tasks. This resource allocation shifts the focus away from the intended action, making it more likely to be forgotten.

Lack of Cues or Reminders

The absence of external prompts can also adversely affect prospective memory. The action may go unexecuted if no cues such as alarms, notes, or even specific environmental landmarks remind the individual of the task. This becomes particularly problematic in complex or busy environments where prospective memory is relied upon for essential tasks.

Aging

As people age, there is often a noticeable decline in cognitive functions, including prospective memory. Age-related cognitive changes can make it more challenging to remember to perform tasks at specific times or contexts. While aging does not necessarily equate to memory loss, it can lead to slower processing speeds and reduced attentional resources. This may manifest as a greater susceptibility to distractions or an increased difficulty retrieving planned actions from memory. Furthermore, the brain's ability to manage multiple tasks concurrently can diminish with age, contributing to lapses in prospective memory.

Prospective Memory Aids

Prospective memory plays a pivotal role in our daily lives, ensuring we remember to execute tasks in the future. It's instrumental in everyday activities such as taking medications, attending appointments, and fulfilling commitments. Yet, like other aspects of memory, prospective memory is prone to errors and lapses.

To counter these lapses, reminders serve as practical tools. Modern technology, especially smartphones and digital assistants, offers a plethora of applications and features to set alarms, send notifications, or even visually represent our upcoming tasks. These technological aids, when coupled with traditional methods like to-do lists or sticky notes, enhance our capacity to remember future tasks.

Additionally, establishing routines can provide a structure that aids memory. For instance, if someone takes their medication after breakfast every day, finishing breakfast can become a cue to take the medicine. Being present or practicing mindfulness can further help. By focusing on the moment, one becomes more aware of one's intentions, plans, and the tasks they set for themselves.

Eyewitness Testimony Errors

Eyewitness testimony errors refer to inaccuracies or mistakes individuals make when providing an account of events they have witnessed, especially in a legal context. These errors can include inaccuracies in identifying suspects, recalling details of the incident, or describing the sequence of events.

Eyewitness testimony errors can occur due to various factors, including stress, leading questioning, the influence of other witnesses, memory decay over time, and issues with cross-racial identification. Such errors can have profound implications for legal proceedings, making it imperative to be aware of eyewitness testimony's potential limitations and fallibility in court.

Eyewitness testimony errors, which can have severe consequences in legal proceedings, are not uncommon. Here are a few examples to illustrate these errors:

- *Mistaken Identity:* In some cases, witnesses may misidentify a suspect during a lineup or in court. For instance, a witness might wrongly identify someone as the perpetrator under stressful conditions, leading to an innocent person's arrest and potential conviction.
- *Inaccurate Recall of Details:* Witnesses might provide inaccurate or inconsistent details about the sequence of events, the appearance of individuals involved, or other critical aspects of a crime. For example, a witness might recall a suspect wearing a red shirt. But, in reality, the shirt was actually blue.
- *Cross-Racial Identification Errors:* Research has shown that people tend to have more difficulty accurately identifying people of a different race than their own. This can lead to misidentification when the witness and suspect belong to other racial or ethnic groups.
- *Memory Contamination:* External factors, such as discussions with other witnesses or exposure to media reports, can influence eyewitnesses. These influences can lead to memory contamination, where a witness incorporates information from others into their account of the events, potentially distorting the accuracy of their testimony.
- *Leading Questions:* During interviews or cross-examinations, attorneys may ask leading questions that suggest specific answers. This can inadvertently influence witnesses to provide responses that align with the attorney's expectations, potentially leading to false or inaccurate testimony.
- *Memory Decay:* Over time, memories can fade or change, making it challenging for witnesses to provide consistent and accurate accounts of events that occurred in the past.

This can result in errors when recalling details or the chronology of an incident.

- **Influence of Stress:** High-stress situations like witnessing a crime can impair memory and lead to errors in recalling key details. Witnesses may experience heightened anxiety, affecting their ability to provide precise and reliable testimony.

Understanding these examples of eyewitness testimony errors underscores the need for caution when relying on such testimony in legal proceedings. Courts and legal professionals must be aware of the potential for these errors and take steps to minimize their impact, such as using unbiased questioning techniques and considering the influence of stress or external factors on witness memory.

Reflections on The Illusion of Memory: Unveiling its Imperfections

Memory stands as a marvel of biological engineering, functioning not only as a repository for storing information but also as a sophisticated system for organizing and reliably retrieving that data. Yet, akin to any intricate biological or technological system, it occasionally exhibits flaws. These momentary lapses in memory can be likened to the intermittent glitches encountered by computer systems when processing vast amounts of information. In the course of daily life, it's common for individuals to experience minor forgetfulness, such as misplacing keys or momentarily struggling to recall a familiar name. These minor lapses are intrinsic to the human condition and typically pose no cause for alarm.

As individuals age, instances of forgetfulness may become more frequent due to natural cognitive changes, including slower processing speed and diminished attention. While some degree of forgetfulness is considered a normal aspect of aging, it's essential to differentiate between these typical lapses and more severe memory impairments that may signal underlying medical or psychological conditions. This distinction is crucial for establishing realistic expectations regarding memory performance and promoting proactive medical intervention when frequent memory lapses disrupt daily functioning or overall well-being.

In instances where memory difficulties persist and significantly impact the quality of life, seeking professional consultation is imperative for accurate diagnosis and appropriate treatment.

CHAPTER 22

Testing Your Memory

Testing your memory is akin to navigating the labyrinth of your mind's intricate corridors. Each memory retrieval task is a meticulous examination of the neural networks at play, providing insights into the resilience or vulnerability of cognitive processes. This scientific endeavor isn't merely a test; it's a diagnostic tool, allowing us to scrutinize the efficiency of your memory to assess cognitive health and unveil potential areas of concern or improvement.

Memory tests are essential tools used by healthcare professionals to assess different aspects of memory function, aiding in the identification of memory impairments, tracking changes over time, and diagnosing memory-related conditions such as Alzheimer's disease or other forms of dementia. These assessments are typically conducted by healthcare professionals with specialized training in neuropsychology, neurology, geriatrics, or psychology. Neuropsychologists, in particular, play a critical role in administering comprehensive memory assessments. They are clinical psychologists with advanced training in evaluating brain-behavior relationships and cognitive function.

During the memory testing process, healthcare professionals administer a battery of tests designed to evaluate various aspects of memory. This assessment usually involves a combination of standardized tests, interviews, observation, and sometimes brain imaging to obtain a comprehensive understanding of an individual's cognitive strengths and weaknesses. By analyzing the test results, tracking changes over time, and developing personalized treatment plans or interventions, these professionals can accurately diagnose memory-related conditions. This approach enables individuals to cope with memory difficulties and improve overall cognitive functioning and quality of life.

Short-Term Memory Tests

These tests assess an individual's ability to temporarily hold and recall a small amount of information over a short period. Suppose you notice changes in your short-term memory abilities; some key short-term memory components may be impacted: capacity, duration, or encoding. Short-term memory tests can help determine if you have a memory problem and which part of short-term memory is responsible. One example of such a test is the Digit Span Test, where the person is asked to repeat a series of digits presented to them in both forward and backward order.

There are several short-term memory assessments available online. These online exams may help you determine if your forgetfulness merits a proper physician examination; however, they should not be the sole tool utilized in diagnosis.

Long-Term Memory Tests

These tests evaluate your ability to remember information from the distant past. Changes in your ability to recall memories from the distant past can be evaluated in a clinical setting to ensure proper diagnosis. Like short-term memory, long-term memory is composed of distinct types: explicit memory, in which information can be recalled consciously, and implicit memory, an umbrella term for the various memories encoded in our unconscious that are not easily accessible by our conscious minds. To account for these differences, testing of long-term memory ability is varied.

For instance, you might be asked by your healthcare provider to recall events from your childhood or historical facts to assess your explicit memory. Implicit memory may be tested instead using evaluations such as word-stem completion tests (patients are given a set of letters and asked to form a complete word; for example: "sim—" could be used to create simple, simile, simultaneous, etc.) or category production tests (patients are given a broad category and asked to list examples of things that would fall into that category, for example: if "fruits" is the given category, banana, apple, and mango would all be acceptable answers).

Sensory Memory Tests

Sensory memory is composed of verbal memory, visual memory, and spatial memory. Our sensory memories depend on our ability to encode information from our outside environment via our senses and subsequently recall that information. Several online examinations may be useful in understanding your ability to encode information that your senses acquire and your ability to retrieve that information later when asked. However, it is important to note that consulting with a healthcare professional is essential for accurate diagnosis and subsequent care planning.

Episodic and Semantic Memory Tests

Episodic memory tests examine your ability to remember specific events or episodes from your life. This type of memory is associated with autobiographical experiences. Episodic memory often overlaps with long-term or short-term memory, so if you are experiencing difficulties recalling events from your life, consider if the events you struggle to recall are typically from your recent memories or more long-term stored memories. Many testing techniques used to analyze episodic memory problems are similar to those used to measure short and long-term memory, such as asking a patient to recall a grocery list or a story.

Semantic memory tests assess an individual's general knowledge and factual information about the world, such as vocabulary, facts, and concepts. This type of memory is commonly tested through a series of verbal fluency assessments. Here, it is important to be mindful of one's first or primary language and the ability to communicate verbally.

The Pyramids and Palms Trees test can be utilized when a verbal assessment is inappropriate. In this nonverbal test, patients are presented with a picture and asked to choose which picture best correlates with the initial image, given two options.

In recent cognitive research, scientists have merged episodic and semantic memory testing based on the assumptions that perception and memory are closely related and that episodic and semantic memory are greatly related. The SEMantic and EPisodic Memory Test (SEMEP) evaluates semantic and episodic memory concurrently through the performance of multiple tasks (naming, recognition, free recall, matching, etc.).

Prospective Memory Tests

These tests evaluate an individual's ability to remember to perform planned actions or tasks in the future, such as remembering to take medication at a specific time. Research shows that prospective memory declines moderately as we age. These changes in prospective memory can be self-reported to a healthcare provider based on self-reporting daily experiences or observations made by family members/caretakers/etc. Or may be diagnosed due to clinical testing.

Scientific literature surrounding prospective memory discusses a supposed "age-prospective memory paradox" in which, in a clinical setting, laboratory-based prospective memory evaluations show more significant memory deficits than self-reported memory concerns. Recent research has shed doubt on this paradox, demonstrating that clinical test results were strongly associated with self-reported measures.

Free Recall Tests

In free recall tests, you are asked to recall as much information as they come from a list or a set of items without any specific order. Unlike pattern identification tasks, free recall tests do not provide any structure or framework to the words being presented, so recall of random words is pinpointed. Several online examinations can be a self-help tool to give a general understanding of your recall abilities. Still, they should not be used in lieu of a healthcare provider's assessment.

Recognition Memory Tests

These tests assess an individual's ability to recognize previously presented information from a list of options. Such tests should be fairly familiar to most of us. Suppose you've ever taken a multiple-choice quiz, for example. In that case, you have completed a recognition memory test on previously studied material.

In the clinical setting, recognition memory is often tested by presenting a patient with a list of words and asking them to study them closely. The learned words are then added randomly throughout a list of new words. The patient is asked to identify which words are from the original list and which are new.

Source Memory Tests

These tests assess an individual's ability to remember the source or context of information, such as where they learned a particular fact. An example would be remembering how you knew there would be a storm on Wednesday by watching the weather channel. The point of source memory is remembering where you got that information from.

Working Memory Tests

These tests evaluate an individual's ability to hold and manipulate information for problem-solving and decision-making temporarily. You can take several online assessments to understand the quality of your working memory, many of which take only a few minutes. A clinical evaluation is always preferable to an online assessment for diagnosing and treating working memory concerns.

Working memory is heavily related to short-term memory. Tests typically focus on one's ability to use short-term memory for problem-solving, processing speed, and reaction time.

Neuropsychological tests, clinical data, and brain imaging form a comprehensive cognitive profile. This data allows for correctly diagnosing and managing brain injuries, stroke, dementia, learning disabilities, and neurological disorders.

These highly specialized tests enable healthcare providers to curate personalized treatment, rehabilitation, and educational strategies to enhance cognitive and functional abilities. As our understanding of various conditions improves and novel cognitive tests are developed, these personalized treatment plans will likely become more effective.

Sensory & Physical Skills Tests

Sensory and physical skills memory testing refers to assessments designed to evaluate an individual's memory and learning abilities related to sensory and motor experiences.

These tests assess how well a person can retain and recall information that involves the senses (sensory memory) and physical movements (motor memory).

The evaluations are often part of neuropsychological assessments to gain insight into how sensory and motor functions interact with memory processes. Some common types of sensory and physical skills memory testing include:

Visual Memory Test

A visual memory test assesses an individual's ability to retain and recall visual information. Participants are typically briefly shown images, patterns, or shapes and then asked to reproduce or recognize them from memory. This test helps evaluate how well a person can retain and recall visual stimuli, which is essential for recognizing faces, reading, and spatial navigation.

Hearing Memory Test

A hearing memory test evaluates an individual's ability to retain and recall auditory information. Participants may be asked to remember a sequence of tones, sounds, or spoken words. This test helps assess the person's auditory memory, which plays an indispensable role in language processing, communication, and memory for spoken information.

Fine Motor Skills Test

A fine motor skills test serves as a comprehensive assessment tool that evaluates an individual's proficiency in controlling and coordinating intricate muscle movements, predominantly focusing on the hands and fingers. During such evaluations, participants may be tasked with a variety of activities, ranging from drawing geometric shapes to writing sentences or even manipulating small objects with precision. Through these tasks, the test offers valuable insights into the individual's manual dexterity and precision, crucial attributes for executing a myriad of everyday activities with accuracy and efficiency.

Whether it's writing legibly, using intricate tools, or performing delicate tasks that demand a high level of precision, fine motor skills are indispensable for navigating daily life effectively. Thus, the outcomes of a fine motor skill test not only provide an indication of an individual's current motor abilities but also offer guidance for interventions aimed at enhancing manual dexterity and overall motor proficiency.

Static Balance Test

A static balance test evaluates an individual's ability to maintain balance and stability while remaining stationary. Participants may be asked to stand on one foot or hold specific postures without swaying or falling.

This test helps assess the person's postural control and ability to stabilize their body, which is key for activities like standing, walking, and maintaining posture during various tasks.

Olfactory and Gustatory Memory Tests

These tests explore the connections between smell, taste, and memory. Our olfactory and gustatory senses are deeply tied to memory recall, as certain scents and flavors can trigger vivid memories. Exercising that involves smelling various scents or identifying tastes can foster stronger memory associations.

Sensory and physical skills tests show promise for memory enhancement. These tests target memory-related brain regions by engaging various senses and movements, leading to improved cognitive performance. As scientific knowledge grows, they may become valuable tools for promoting cognitive vitality and preserving memory throughout life.

Brain Imaging Tests

Brain imaging tests are medical procedures that allow healthcare professionals to visualize and examine the brain's structure, function, and activity.

These tests provide valuable information about brain health and can aid in diagnosing various neurological conditions and disorders. Brain imaging tests may be used for memory problems in specific situations where there is a need to rule out or investigate underlying neurological conditions that could be contributing to memory issues.

While memory problems can have various causes, some of which may not require brain imaging, using brain imaging tests can be helpful under the following circumstances:

1. *Unexplained or Severe Memory Loss:* When an individual experiences severe or unexplained memory loss, brain imaging tests can be valuable in identifying potential structural abnormalities in the brain, such as tumors, strokes, or lesions.

2. *Early-Onset Memory Problems:* If memory problems are present in relatively young individuals (below the age of 65), brain imaging tests may be considered to assess for rare causes of cognitive decline, such as early-onset Alzheimer's disease or other neurodegenerative disorders.

3. *Progressive Memory Decline:* If memory problems progressively worsen over time, brain imaging can help identify any degenerative changes in the brain that could contribute to the decline.

4. *History of Head Trauma:* In cases where memory problems are associated with a history of head trauma, brain imaging can help detect structural brain damage or evidence of traumatic brain injury.

5. *Assessment for Dementia:* When memory problems are suspected to be related to dementia or other progressive cognitive disorders, brain imaging can provide additional evidence to support the diagnosis and determine the extent of brain changes.

6. *Identifying Treatable Conditions:* Sometimes, memory problems may be caused by treatable conditions like brain infections or tumors. Brain imaging can help detect these conditions early for appropriate intervention.

The decision to use brain imaging tests for memory problems should be made by healthcare professionals based on the individual's medical history, symptoms, and clinical presentation. The goal is to ensure accurate diagnosis, appropriate management, and the best possible care for the individual experiencing memory difficulties. Some brain imaging tools that can be utilized to diagnose and identify brain conditions include:

Computed Tomography (CT) Scan

A CT scan uses X-rays to create detailed cross-sectional images of the brain. Brain CT scans can be helpful in the clinical setting to understand why memory problems might occur and provide a framework for healthcare providers to structure care and treatment. Suppose a CT scan reveals shrinkage of regional brain matter or a blood clot blocking oxygen supply to a brain region.

In that case, your healthcare provider may suggest further investigating dementia. Suppose a CT scan reveals a tumor, infection, or skull fracture. However, other diagnoses and treatment plans will likely be discussed in that case. Overall, this technology helps detect abnormalities and inform practical next steps in the clinical setting.

Magnetic Resonance Imaging (MRI)

MRI uses powerful magnets and radio waves to produce detailed images of the brain's soft tissues. Like CT scans, this technology is incredibly valuable in the clinical setting for understanding the cause of memory problems and allowing for proper diagnosis of conditions. MRI technology effectively visualizes brain structures and identifies abnormalities like tumors, strokes, and multiple sclerosis lesions. Repeated MRIs can show disease progression in cases of neurodegenerative dementia.

Functional Magnetic Resonance Imaging (fMRI)

fMRI measures brain activity by detecting changes in blood flow. It is commonly used in research and clinical settings to study brain function related to memory, language, emotion, and various cognitive processes. This technology is instrumental in diagnosing vascular dementia.

Diffusion Tensor Imaging (DTI)

DTI is a type of MRI that examines the brain's white matter tracts. DTI detects water diffusion in the brain's white matter. This technology provides healthcare providers with information about the integrity and connectivity of brain pathways. It is used to study conditions like traumatic brain injury and white matter diseases. These images allow for brain mapping, which allows for a greater understanding of the connectivity within an individual's brain, especially before any invasive procedures.

Positron Emission Tomography (PET) Scan

PET scans use radioactive tracers to measure brain activity and metabolism. It is often used to assess brain function and detect areas of abnormal activity, such as epilepsy or certain types of dementia. Amyloid PET scans are a specific type of scan that tags the beta-amyloid protein to ascertain the level of beta-amyloid protein in the brain. Elevated beta-amyloid levels may be indicative of amyloid-beta plaques. Healthcare providers can utilize amyloid PET scans to diagnose Alzheimer's disease, a condition associated with amyloid plaques on the brain.

Single-Photon Emission Computed Tomography (SPECT) Scan

SPECT is another nuclear imaging technique that uses radioactive tracers to assess blood flow and brain activity. It is often used to evaluate brain function and detect abnormalities related to seizures, brain injuries, and other neurological disorders. SPECT scans are controversial in the medical community. This technology is not available outside of health centers operated by the inventor— Dr. Daniel Amen. Only his facilities are equipped to perform and read these tests, making it a controversial practice for the rest of the neurological community. The reported benefits of SPECT scans are highly variable. Most institutions or clinics will not prescribe this testing if you seek medical treatment for memory loss.

Brain imaging tests are not usually the first-line assessment for memory problems. A comprehensive clinical evaluation and neuropsychological testing often suffice to identify the cause. Brain imaging is reserved for cases with specific clinical indications or suspicion of underlying neurological conditions that require further investigation.

Spinal Fluid Tests

Spinal fluid tests, also known as cerebrospinal fluid (CSF) tests, are not typically used as a routine or first-line assessment for memory problems. Instead, they are primarily employed in specific situations where certain neurological conditions are suspected, or other diagnostic methods have not provided a definitive diagnosis. These tests are generally considered when there is a need to investigate potential underlying causes of memory problems involving the central nervous system.

Here are some situations where spinal fluid tests might be considered for memory problems:

1. ***Ruling out Infections:*** Spinal fluid tests can help rule out central nervous system infections, such as bacterial or viral meningitis or encephalitis. In some cases, certain infections may lead to memory problems as a symptom.

2. ***Assessing Inflammatory Conditions:*** CSF analysis can identify inflammation markers, which might indicate conditions like autoimmune disorders affecting the nervous system. Some inflammatory conditions can cause cognitive impairment, including memory problems.

3. ***Diagnosing Certain Neurological Disorders:*** Spinal fluid tests can be used to assist in diagnosing certain neurological conditions that may be causing memory problems, such as Creutzfeldt-Jakob disease or other prion diseases.

4. ***Detecting Markers of Neurodegeneration:*** In specific cases where there is a concern about neurodegenerative diseases like Alzheimer's or other forms of dementia, spinal fluid tests may be used to look for particular biomarkers associated with these conditions.

5. ***Exploring Rare Neurological Causes:*** For some with early-onset memory problems or atypical cognitive symptoms, spinal fluid tests may be considered to investigate rare neurological causes that might not be apparent through other diagnostic methods.

Spinal fluid tests are invasive and not routine for memory problems. They are considered if other evaluations are inconclusive or if specific neurological conditions are suspected. Decisions are made case-by-case, so discussing benefits, risks, and implications with your doctor is essential.

Many of these emerging therapies are still early in research and clinical trials. While they offer hope for future treatments, further investigation is needed to determine their safety, effectiveness, and long-term outcomes. As our understanding of the brain continues to evolve, these innovative approaches may revolutionize how we address memory problems and enhance brain health. As the field of neuroscience continues to evolve, it is expected that more innovative and personalized approaches to memory loss treatment will emerge, providing new avenues of hope for people affected by this challenging condition.

Reflections on Testing Your Memory

Memory testing is not just a simple evaluation of one's ability to recall information but rather a captivating journey into the depths of the mind. It's like exploring a vast and intricate labyrinth, where each memory test is a turn in the maze, revealing new insights into the intricate workings of the cognitive landscape.

From standardized tests to online assessments, the options for memory testing are vast and varied. Each test offers a distinctive approach, testing different facets of memory, from visual recall to verbal memory and working memory. Moreover, researchers are continually developing innovative ways to explore the complexities of memory, from using virtual reality to creating immersive memory tests to utilizing neuroimaging techniques to investigate the neural underpinnings of memory.

At the heart of memory testing lies a profound reflection on one's recollections. It's not just about what you remember but how you remember it. Each test invites introspection, inviting you to analyze your thought processes and cognitive patterns. By engaging in memory testing, you embark on a transformative process of self-discovery, uncovering the unique tapestry of experiences and knowledge that forms the basis of your memories.

Memory testing is empowering. It enables you to assess your cognitive strengths and weaknesses, empowering you to adopt strategies to enhance your memory function. With each test, you gain valuable insights into the malleability of your mind, unlocking new avenues for cognitive growth and enrichment.

In essence, memory testing is a voyage of self-exploration, an opportunity to engage with the complexities of the mind and emerge with a deeper understanding of one's cognitive identity. It's an ongoing journey, filled with twists and turns, that ultimately leads to a more profound appreciation of the intricate relationship between the past, present, and future in shaping our memories.

CHAPTER 23

When to See a Doctor

When the threads of memory start to fray, consulting a doctor becomes the proactive step toward cognitive well-being. If you forget important details or face persistent confusion, it's time to bring in a medical ally. Memory problems are complex puzzles, and seeking professional guidance offers personalized solutions. Your brain deserves the best care, and a doctor specializing in memory concerns can be the guiding light toward preserving and enhancing its functionality.

Navigating the maze of life with a foggy memory can be frustrating, bewildering, and downright scary. You might forget names, misplace items, or blank out during conversations. While everyone experiences occasional memory lapses, when forgetfulness begins to interfere with your daily life, it's time to consult a healthcare professional. This isn't just another thing to tick off your to-do list; it's a vital step in safeguarding your mental health and overall well-being.

Why should you see a doctor? Because forgetting things might be a small warning sign of more significant health issues hiding below the surface. This could mean problems with your brain, issues with your hormones, or even something as serious as Alzheimer's disease that could change your life. Catching these problems early by talking to a doctor can make it easier to treat them quickly. If you wait too long, it could make things much harder to deal with later.

Once you take that step into the medical office, you're not just getting a diagnosis—you're opening a gateway to a world of options specifically designed to improve your life. The healthcare provider becomes your partner, collaboratively working with you to develop a tailor-made strategy that could involve a myriad of treatments, therapies, and coping skills. We're talking about a custom-built arsenal aimed at helping you navigate the daily intricacies of life more easily.

The value of a thorough medical assessment cannot be overstated. It's not just about labeling your condition; it's about identifying the root cause of your memory issues, be it stress, hormone imbalance, or something far more severe. Once the bullseye is identified, you can take aim with targeted interventions. Imagine being handed a GPS that directs you through the labyrinthine world of medical treatments right to the therapies that are designed to work for you.

You have lots of choices for treatment. You could get medicine that helps your brain work better, make changes in your life to feel more in control, do brain exercises to think more clearly, or even try different therapies that treat your whole self, not just your memory. The best part is the plan is made just for you. It's not a one-size-fits-all treatment; it's your own special path to feeling better.

In sum, visiting a healthcare professional for memory issues isn't just a preventative measure. It's a transformative journey that could dramatically improve your quality of life. By catching problems early and crafting a personalized game plan, you equip yourself with the tools to live more fully, mindfully, and happily. And who doesn't want that?

A visit to a primary physician is the first step. If any of the following symptoms are present, a referral is conducted if the following are present:

1. *Early Detection of Underlying Conditions:* Memory problems can sometimes be like the smoke that signals a hidden fire. They can indicate deeper health problems like Alzheimer's, dementia, thyroid issues, vitamin deficiencies, or infections. Catching these issues in their early stages could be a game-changer. You'll have more options for treatment and a better chance of slowing down or managing the condition effectively. It's like nipping the problem in the bud before it grows into a much bigger, harder-to-control issue.

2. *Proper Diagnosis:* Think of a healthcare professional as your personal detective for health. They don't just look at the surface; they dig deep. They'll conduct detailed tests on your cognitive functions, review your past medical history, and may even order lab tests or brain scans. This comprehensive review is Important because it pinpoints the exact reason behind your memory problems, ensuring you don't waste time or resources on the wrong treatment.

3. *Treatment Options:* Once you have a precise diagnosis, it's like having a roadmap for how to get better. Treatments can be as varied as the conditions they aim to cure. Alzheimer's has specific medications to help slow its progression when caught early. If you're facing vitamin

deficiencies, a simple diet change or supplements can turn things around. The beauty of having options is that they empower you to control your health.

4. **Medication Management:** Sometimes, the cure becomes the curse. If you're already on medication for other conditions, those drugs might be causing or worsening your memory issues. Your doctor can review your current medications and adjust the dosages or switch you to an alternative that is less likely to affect your cognitive functions. This way, you continue treating your original medical issue without the unwanted side effect of memory loss.

5. **Lifestyle Recommendations:** Often, the way we live our daily lives can be the unsung hero or villain in our health story. Your healthcare provider can guide you toward lifestyle changes that positively impact your brain health. Imagine customizing your diet to include more brain-boosting nutrients or establishing an exercise routine that keeps you fit and sharpens your mind. Stress management techniques and cognitive exercises could be added to your daily regimen to keep your brain as fit as your body.

6. **Emotional Support:** Memory issues can be emotionally draining, leading to feelings of frustration, sadness, or anxiety. Your healthcare provider is well-equipped to offer you medical and emotional support. They can refer you to support groups or counseling services specializing in helping people with memory-related emotional challenges. It's like having a safety net of emotional support to catch you when you fall.

7. **Monitoring and Follow-Up:** Your journey doesn't end with a single doctor's appointment; it's more like a continuous loop. Regular check-ups are vital to monitor the effectiveness of your treatment. If something isn't working or there are new developments, your treatment plan can be quickly tweaked to suit your needs. It's a way to stay one step ahead of your condition.

8. **Peace of Mind:** Taking proactive steps to address your memory issues is an emotional stabilizer for you and your loved ones. It can significantly reduce the cloud of worry that often accompanies health problems. This peace of mind can be invaluable, leading to a better quality of life, less stress, and a more optimistic outlook.

If you or someone you care about is dealing with memory issues, it's essential to go see a doctor. Getting the right medical help can give you an accurate understanding of what's causing the problem, how to treat it, and how to manage it over time.

Taking early steps to address these issues can make a big difference in keeping your mind sharp and preserving your mental skills. So don't wait—get a thorough check-up from a healthcare professional and a personalized plan to manage the issue.

Reflections on When to See a Doctor

The decision of when to see a doctor unfolds as an essential chapter in the narrative of self-care and well-being. It's akin to recognizing the signs on the journey of your own health story, where intuition and awareness become guiding lights in navigating the human body's complexities.

Knowing when to seek medical advice is not merely a matter of physical symptoms; it's an acknowledgment of the intricate dialogue between your body and mind.

Consider this decision as tuning into your body's unique language. It's an understanding that your body communicates through symptoms, urging you to interpret its signals. Whether it's a sudden onset of symptoms or the persistence of discomfort, your body's messages become cues guiding you to the healthcare chapter of your story.

Moreover, recognizing when to seek medical advice is an act of self-advocacy—acknowledging that your health narrative matters and your well-being deserves attention. This decision is not just about addressing acute issues but also about preventive care, creating a narrative of proactive health management.

In the grand tapestry of your health story, deciding when to see a doctor becomes a pivotal plot point. It reflects self-awareness, a willingness to listen to your body's narrative, and an empowered step towards prioritizing your health. As you navigate this journey, remember that seeking medical advice is not just about addressing ailments but about fostering a holistic narrative of well-being.

CHAPTER 24

Navigating Dementia's Challenges

Exploring the intricate landscape of dementia, with its widespread impact, reveals a dynamic challenge affecting cognition and daily life. Beyond medical aspects, societal hurdles include isolation fueled by stigmas. Humanitarian efforts aim to erase these stigmas through empathy and community involvement. A comprehensive understanding, from diverse manifestations to prevention strategies, is vital for informed clinical practices and supportive community bonds.

The urgency of understanding what causes dementia is amplified by its widespread impact and growing prevalence. As a progressive condition affecting cognitive function, behavior, and daily living activities, dementia currently afflicts over 78 million people worldwide—a figure expected to triple by 2050. While not a single disease, dementia is a complex collection of symptoms that impact memory, thinking, and social skills.

As the seventh leading cause of death globally, it presents a public health crisis that demands medical experts, policymakers, and communities' attention. Although no cure exists, various treatments can help manage its debilitating symptoms. Those concerned about cognitive decline should seek medical advice for accurate diagnosis and appropriate treatment plans.

The societal impact of dementia extends beyond medical considerations, often leading to isolation and misunderstanding due to associated stigmas. Humanitarian efforts in this area focus on destigmatizing the condition through empathy and recognizing the individual's unique experiences and aspirations.

Community involvement, including support groups and volunteer initiatives, significantly enhances the quality of life for those affected by dementia. Understanding the disease comprehensively—from its types, symptoms, and risk factors to its diagnostic methods, treatments, and prevention strategies—provides a nuanced view that can inform clinical practice and community support.

Types of Dementia

Dementia is not a single disease but a term that describes symptoms impairing cognitive functions such as memory, thinking, and reasoning. Its various types present different challenges and symptoms and require diverse treatment approaches.

- *Alzheimer's Disease:* As the most prevalent form of dementia, Alzheimer's Disease accounts for 60-80% of all dementia cases. It is characterized by memory loss, confusion, and difficulty performing daily tasks. The disease primarily targets the brain's hippocampus, affecting memory and learning capabilities.
- *Vascular Dementia:* Often occurring after a stroke, Vascular Dementia results from impaired blood flow to the brain. Symptoms can be sudden or gradual, including impaired judgment, difficulty planning, and reduced concentration. It emphasizes the vital link between cardiovascular health and cognitive function.
- *Lewy Body Dementia (LBD):* Representing 6.9% of dementia cases, LBD is caused by the abnormal accumulation of protein deposits known as Lewy bodies. Individuals with LBD may experience visual hallucinations, motor symptoms similar to Parkinson's Disease, and fluctuating cognitive abilities.
- *Frontotemporal Dementia:* Making up 3.3% of dementia cases, this type targets the frontal and temporal lobes of the brain. It often leads to drastic personality changes, difficulty with language, and complex thinking problems.
- *Creutzfeldt-Jakob Disease (CJD):* A rare and rapidly progressive neurodegenerative disorder that manifests with a variety of unique symptoms. This disease is characterized by cognitive decline, leading to profound dementia and neurological symptoms such as muscle stiffness, twitching, and weakness. Unlike other forms of dementia, CJD typically progresses at a rapid pace, often within a year of symptom onset.
- *Mixed Dementia:* The coexistence of Alzheimer's Disease with other forms of dementia, such as Vascular Dementia or LBD. Mixed dementia highlights the complexity of diagnosis, as symptoms overlap, making it challenging to determine the precise type.

- **Reversible Dementias:** Some rare types of dementia, such as those caused by vitamin deficiencies or thyroid issues, may be reversible with proper treatment. These cases underscore the importance of early and accurate diagnosis.

The many faces of dementia reveal a complex landscape of cognitive disorders that manifest in many ways. Each type presents unique characteristics and requires tailored care and treatment strategies. Early diagnosis and targeted interventions can significantly improve the quality of life for individuals with dementia and their families. A comprehensive understanding of these various types is fundamental for healthcare providers, caregivers, and society to approach dementia with empathy, efficiency, and effectiveness.

What Causes Dementia?

Dementia is not merely a medical term; it is a poignant reality that affects the lives of millions across the globe. A word synonymous with fear, confusion, and often misunderstanding, dementia refers to a broad category of brain diseases. But what causes dementia? What unseen processes within the brain and body lead to this severe decline in cognitive function?

While most associate dementia with aging, the truth is far more complex. Multiple factors, from genetics and neurological changes to environmental exposures and lifestyle choices, weave a multifaceted tapestry that defines an individual's risk of developing dementia. The most common causes of dementia include:

- **Genetic Factors:** Genetics play a role in certain types of dementia, such as Alzheimer's disease. While having specific genes may increase the risk, it does not guarantee the development of the condition. Familial Alzheimer's, caused by gene mutations, is rare but leads to early-onset dementia.
- **Age and Neurological Changes:** Aging is the most significant risk factor for dementia, especially after 65 years of age. Neurological changes in the brain that occur with aging may lead to atrophy and reduced cognitive function.
- **Vascular Conditions:** Vascular dementia results from conditions affecting the blood vessels, reducing blood flow to the brain. Strokes, atherosclerosis, and other vascular issues may contribute to this type of dementia.

- *Lifestyle Choices and Environmental Factors:* Poor lifestyle choices such as excessive alcohol consumption, smoking, lack of exercise, and an unhealthy diet can increase the risk of dementia. Exposure to certain environmental toxins has also been associated with a heightened risk.
- *Brain Injuries and Trauma:* Traumatic brain injuries and repeated head trauma can cause specific types of dementia. Former athletes involved in contact sports or individuals with a history of severe accidents may be at higher risk.
- *Chronic Diseases:* Chronic health conditions such as diabetes, hypertension, obesity, and heart disease can all contribute to the risk of developing dementia.
- *Mental Health and Social Engagement:* Depression and social isolation may have a role in the development of dementia. Engaging in mental and social activities is often seen as protective.

The causes of dementia are numerous and complex, with a unique interplay between genetic, biological, environmental, and lifestyle factors. This condition has no single cause, making prevention and treatment a multifaceted challenge.

Understanding these underlying factors is central to advancing research, improving diagnosis, and creating targeted interventions to delay or prevent dementia.

Early Warnings and Symptoms of Dementia

Understanding the symptoms of dementia, particularly the early warnings and how the condition progresses, is key for timely diagnosis, intervention, and care. These are the early warning signs of dementia, the progression of symptoms, and unique symptoms for different types of dementia:

- *Memory Loss:* One of the most frequently observed early signs of dementia. It often manifests as forgetfulness, particularly regarding newly acquired information. Individuals may be unable to remember important dates, conversations, or tasks.
- *Difficulty with Language and Communication:* Individuals may struggle with finding the right words during conversations, leading to noticeable pauses or incomplete sentences. They might also repeat themselves or

have difficulty following the thread of a conversation or participating meaningfully in it.

- ***Trouble with Complex Tasks:*** Tasks that require planning, organization, or problem-solving become increasingly challenging. For example, someone may find it difficult to follow a familiar recipe, manage finances, or remember the rules of a game they used to enjoy.
- ***Confusion about Time and Place:*** There's a loss of sense of time and an increasing disorientation regarding dates and the passage of time. This may manifest as missing appointments, forgetting the day of the week, or becoming confused about their location.
- ***Misplacing Things:*** Items are frequently put in odd or inappropriate places. Unlike ordinary forgetfulness, individuals often cannot retrace their steps to locate the misplaced items, causing increased stress and frustration.
- ***Poor Judgment:*** Decision-making skills deteriorate, which can lead to inappropriate or risky behavior. Examples include poor financial decisions like giving away large sums of money to strangers or making hasty purchases.
- ***Withdrawal from Social Activities:*** People may lose interest in hobbies, social gatherings, and other activities that used to bring them joy. This withdrawal is often due to a combination of cognitive decline and decreased self-confidence.

Recognizing the early warnings and symptoms of dementia is Important for timely intervention and care. Understanding the progression of symptoms and the unique manifestations of different types of dementia aids in providing appropriate support and improving the quality of life for individuals and their families.

If you observe these signs, seeking medical advice and support early on can make a significant difference in managing the condition effectively. Stay informed, stay vigilant, and foster a compassionate environment to navigate the challenges posed by dementia with empathy and understanding.

Dementia Progression Stages

Dementia encompasses a spectrum of stages, each marked by unique symptoms and complexities. From the initial subtle indicators to the advanced challenges in daily life, the progression unfolds in distinct phases. Understanding these stages is essential for tailoring effective care strategies and support for individuals and their caregivers navigating the intricate landscape of dementia.

1. ***Mild Stage:*** At this initial phase, the impact of memory issues becomes more noticeable, extending its reach into daily life activities. The individual may encounter challenges in remembering recent events, and skills related to problem-solving and planning may exhibit a subtle decline. These changes can subtly erode the sense of independence as cognitive functions gradually wane.

2. ***Moderate Stage:*** Progressing into the moderate stage, the symptoms take on a more pronounced and challenging nature. Forgetfulness intensifies, affecting not only recent events but also making recognition of familiar faces and places increasingly difficult. Emotional shifts, such as heightened irritability, anxiety, or depression, add an additional layer of complexity to the individual's experience, impacting both their own well-being and interactions with others.

3. ***Severe Stage:*** As dementia reaches its advanced phase, comprehensive and continuous care becomes imperative. Communication becomes severely limited, with the individual struggling to express thoughts or understand language. The decline in physical capabilities is profound, rendering even basic tasks like eating or dressing challenging. The need for around-the-clock care underscores the profound impact of the disease on both cognitive and physical functioning, emphasizing the critical role of support during this demanding stage.

Unique Symptoms for Different Types of Dementia

Dementia is a broad term covering various conditions, and recognizing the distinct symptoms associated with each type is essential for precise diagnosis and tailored care. Different types of dementia manifest with unique cognitive, behavioral, and physical characteristics, allowing healthcare professionals to differentiate between them and provide appropriate interventions.

Alzheimer's Disease

Alzheimer's Disease is characterized by distinctive symptoms, most notably significant memory loss, primarily affecting recent events. Individuals with Alzheimer's often face challenges in problem-solving, planning, and completing familiar tasks independently. Another prominent feature is confusion regarding time and place, a hallmark of this type of dementia. As the disease progresses, individuals may experience difficulty in recognizing familiar faces, including those of close family members. Additionally, language difficulties may arise, affecting the ability to express thoughts and understand conversations. Behavioral changes such as mood swings, withdrawal, or changes in personality are common.

Vascular Dementia

Vascular Dementia presents a distinct set of symptoms associated with impaired blood flow to the brain. The hallmark of this condition is difficulties with reasoning, judgment, and problem-solving. Individuals may experience challenges in planning and organizing tasks, impacting their ability to carry out daily activities. Memory loss is common, but it often involves difficulty recalling recent events rather than a significant overall decline. Additionally, individuals with Vascular Dementia may exhibit fluctuations in alertness and concentration. Speech and language difficulties, such as trouble finding the right words or understanding speech, may arise.

Physical symptoms can include gait disturbances, with individuals having difficulty walking or maintaining balance. The onset of symptoms is often abrupt, especially after a stroke or a series of small strokes.

Lewy Body Dementia

Lewy Body Dementia (LBD) exhibits distinctive symptoms that differentiate it from other forms of dementia. Key features include fluctuating cognitive abilities, visual hallucinations, and motor symptoms similar to Parkinson's disease, such as tremors and rigidity. Individuals with LBD often experience vivid and recurring hallucinations that may contribute to confusion and distress.

Fluctuations in alertness and attention, termed "fluctuating cognition," are common, leading to variations in the individual's ability to engage in daily activities. Additionally, LBD may cause rapid eye movement (REM) sleep behavior disorder, resulting in physically acting out dreams during sleep. Other symptoms encompass autonomic dysfunction, affecting blood pressure regulation, digestion, and temperature control. Delusions and paranoia may also occur in some cases.

Frontotemporal Dementia

Frontotemporal Dementia (FTD) exhibits distinctive symptoms primarily affecting the frontal and temporal lobes of the brain, leading to changes in behavior, personality, and language skills. Behavioral changes may manifest as socially inappropriate actions, apathy, loss of empathy, or repetitive behaviors. Alterations in personality can include a lack of inhibition, impulsivity, or rigid thinking.

Language difficulties are prevalent, with individuals experiencing challenges in expressing or understanding speech, and some may exhibit echolalia (a linguistic phenomenon characterized by the automatic and involuntary repetition of vocalizations or sounds). Memory and spatial skills usually remain relatively intact in the early stages, distinguishing FTD from other forms of dementia.

The specific symptoms can vary based on the subtype of FTD, such as behavioral variant FTD, semantic variant primary progressive aphasia (svPPA), and nonfluent variant primary progressive aphasia (nfvPPA).

Creutzfeldt-Jakob Disease (CJD)

Creutzfeldt-Jakob Disease (CJD) is characterized by distinct and rapidly progressing symptoms that set it apart from other neurological conditions. The most prominent feature is a swift decline in cognitive functions, including memory, thinking, and reasoning abilities, surpassing typical age-related cognitive changes. Patients often exhibit muscle stiffness, twitching, and weakness, leading to a loss of coordination. As the disease advances, individuals may lose the ability to move purposefully and articulate coherent speech.

Behavioral changes, such as mood alterations, depression, and anxiety, are common, accompanied by personality shifts. Visual disturbances, including blurred vision, may also manifest due to the impact on neurological functions. It's important to recognize that different forms of CJD, including sporadic, familial, iatrogenic, and variant, can present with varied symptoms. Diagnosis involves a comprehensive approach, including clinical evaluation, brain imaging, cerebrospinal fluid testing, and, occasionally, a brain biopsy. While there is no cure for CJD, treatment focuses on managing symptoms and providing supportive care.

In summary, each type of dementia necessitates tailored care strategies to address the specific challenges associated with its distinct set of symptoms. Tailoring care strategies involves a comprehensive understanding of the individual's unique symptoms, preferences, and stage of dementia. This personalized approach enhances the effectiveness of care, improving the individual's quality of life and providing support that aligns with their specific needs and challenges. Moreover, involving healthcare professionals, caregivers, and support networks ensures a holistic and collaborative approach to dementia care, addressing the multifaceted aspects of the condition for the well-being of the affected individuals and their families.

Psychological Symptoms for Most Types of Dementia

Dementia encompasses a broad spectrum of neurodegenerative disorders characterized by cognitive decline and impairment in multiple domains of mental functioning. While the specific symptoms may vary depending on the type and stage of dementia, there are several psychological symptoms commonly associated with most forms of dementia:

- *Memory Loss:* One of the hallmark features of dementia is progressive memory loss, particularly affecting recent memories. Individuals may have difficulty recalling recent events, conversations, or information.
- *Confusion and Disorientation:* Dementia often leads to confusion about time, place, and people. Individuals may become disoriented and have trouble recognizing familiar surroundings or people, even in familiar environments.
- *Impaired Judgment and Decision-Making:* Dementia can impair an individual's ability to make sound judgments and decisions. They may struggle with tasks requiring complex reasoning or planning.
- *Difficulty with Language and Communication:* Many people with dementia experience difficulty finding the right words, following conversations, or understanding speech. Expressive language may also become impaired, leading to difficulty in articulating thoughts or ideas.
- *Changes in Mood and Personality:* Dementia can cause significant changes in mood and behavior. Individuals may experience mood swings, irritability, agitation, or apathy. Personality changes, such as increased impulsivity or social withdrawal, may also occur.

- **Depression and Anxiety:** Depression and anxiety are common psychological symptoms in individuals with dementia. Feelings of sadness, hopelessness, or worry may be exacerbated by the challenges of coping with cognitive decline.
- **Psychosis:** Some individuals with dementia may experience hallucinations (seeing or hearing things that are not there) or delusions (false beliefs). These symptoms can be distressing for both the individual and their caregivers.
- **Sleep Disturbances:** Changes in sleep patterns are common in dementia, with individuals experiencing disruptions in sleep-wake cycles, insomnia, or excessive daytime sleepiness.
- **Agitation and Aggression:** In some cases, dementia can lead to agitation, restlessness, or aggressive behavior. This may manifest as verbal or physical outbursts, especially when the individual feels confused or frustrated.
- **Wandering and Repetitive Behaviors:** Individuals with dementia may engage in wandering or repetitive behaviors, such as pacing, searching for familiar objects, or asking the same questions repeatedly.

It's important to note that the presentation and severity of psychological symptoms can vary widely among individuals with dementia. Additionally, certain types of dementia may have specific symptom profiles or patterns of progression. Prompt diagnosis and appropriate management of these symptoms are essential for optimizing the quality of life for individuals living with dementia and their caregivers.

Risk Factors in Dementia

The risk factors for dementia vary across conditions, such as Alzheimer's disease, vascular dementia, Lewy body dementia, and all other types. Understanding these risk factors is essential in taking proactive measures to prevent or delay the onset of dementia. Here are some of the prominent risk factors associated with dementia:

- **Age:** Age is one of the most significant risk factors for dementia. The likelihood of developing this cognitive disorder escalates notably for those above the age of 65. As people continue to age, this risk becomes even more pronounced. Older age groups, particularly those in their 80s and 90s, have a higher incidence of dementia.

- *Genetics and Family History:* While not all forms of dementia are hereditary, genetics can play a role, especially in specific types such as Alzheimer's disease. Having a close family member with dementia can also suggest a higher risk, although it's important to note that many people with a family history never develop the condition themselves.
- *Cardiovascular Health:* Factors that negatively affect cardiovascular health, such as high blood pressure, elevated cholesterol levels, obesity, and diabetes, can also increase the risk of dementia. Such health issues may lead to vascular dementia, which is caused by impaired blood flow to the brain, thereby affecting cognitive function.
- *Head Injuries:* Traumatic brain injuries (TBI), especially if they are repeated or severe, have been linked to a greater risk of developing dementia later in life. These injuries may cause structural damage to the brain or accelerate the deposition of abnormal proteins, contributing to cognitive decline.
- *Mental and Social Engagement:* A lifestyle that lacks mental stimulation or social interaction can make an individual more susceptible to dementia. Engaging in activities that challenge the brain, such as reading, puzzles, or learning new skills, as well as maintaining an active social life, may provide some degree of protective benefit against dementia.
- *Substance Abuse:* Chronic abuse of substances like alcohol and tobacco has been associated with a heightened risk of dementia. Both smoking and excessive alcohol consumption have detrimental effects on vascular health, which can, in turn, impact cognitive abilities.
- *Depression:* Although the relationship between depression and dementia is not fully understood, studies suggest that depression might be a potential risk factor. It is unclear whether depression is a precursor to dementia, a symptom of cognitive decline, or if both conditions share common underlying mechanisms.
- *Education:* Lower formal education levels correlate with a higher risk of developing dementia. The theory behind this is that higher education might expose individuals to a range

of mentally stimulating activities throughout their lives, thereby offering some cognitive resilience.

Various chronic conditions, such as Parkinson's disease and HIV, can heighten the susceptibility to specific forms of dementia. While factors like age and genetics remain beyond our influence, proactive measures can be taken to manage other risk factors. Prioritizing cardiovascular health, making positive lifestyle choices, and adopting a healthy overall lifestyle contribute to risk reduction.

Engaging in mental and social activities, coupled with effective management of chronic health conditions, forms an important approach to diminishing the likelihood of dementia. This not only facilitates targeted prevention strategies but also allows for early interventions, significantly influencing the lives of individuals at risk of encountering this complex and life-altering condition.

How Doctors Determine Dementia

Diagnosing dementia is a complex process that requires careful consideration of various factors and symptoms. The condition can manifest in several ways, and its underlying causes can be multifaceted, making accurate diagnosis challenging. Here's an exploration of how doctors typically determine dementia through various diagnostic techniques:

- *Medical History and Physical Examination:* The diagnosis of dementia generally commences with an exhaustive review of the patient's medical history, coupled with a physical examination. Doctors look for clues about cognitive or neurological symptoms' onset, duration, and progression. They may also delve into family history concerning dementia or other neurological conditions. Additionally, underlying health issues, such as cardiovascular diseases that might contribute to cognitive deficits, are considered.

- *Cognitive and Neuropsychological Tests:* This stage involves a series of tests aimed at gauging cognitive faculties like memory, problem-solving capabilities, attention span, language skills, and other aspects of mental function. A frequently used test is the Mini-Mental State Examination (MMSE), designed to give clinicians a snapshot of a patient's cognitive health and identify any irregularities.

- **Laboratory Tests:** Blood and other lab-based diagnostics help rule out alternative explanations for cognitive issues, such as thyroid problems or vitamin deficiencies. These tests can confirm or eliminate other potential causes of the symptoms, aiding in a more accurate diagnosis.

- **Brain Imaging:** Various imaging techniques, like Magnetic Resonance Imaging (MRI) or Computed Tomography (CT) scans, may be used to visualize the brain's structure. These scans can reveal any abnormalities, such as tumors or signs of stroke, which could be contributing to the symptoms. Positron Emission Tomography (PET) scans are also used to visualize amyloid plaques in the brain, a characteristic feature of Alzheimer's disease.

- **Psychiatric Evaluation:** As symptoms of dementia can overlap with those of other psychiatric conditions like depression, a comprehensive psychiatric assessment is often needed. This helps differentiate dementia from other disorders and can be fundamental for developing a tailored treatment plan.

- **Assessment of Daily Functioning:** A key part of the diagnostic process is evaluating how the symptoms affect the patient's day-to-day life. This might include assessing the person's ability to undertake daily activities such as cooking, maintaining personal hygiene, and managing finances. It helps healthcare providers understand the level of impairment and plan appropriate interventions.

- **Specialist Referral:** In instances where the diagnosis is challenging or requires specialized expertise, a referral to a neurologist, geriatrician, or another specialist well-versed in dementia may be recommended. These professionals can offer more detailed assessments and advanced diagnostic tests.

- **Ongoing Monitoring:** Diagnosing dementia can be an evolving process. This is especially true in the early stages, where symptoms may be subtle or easily confused with normal aging or other conditions. Therefore, regular follow-up appointments and continuous monitoring are typically necessary to confirm the diagnosis and track the disease's progression.

Diagnosing dementia is a multifaceted process requiring clinical evaluation, cognitive testing, laboratory investigation, and imaging studies. The goal is not only to identify dementia but also to pinpoint its type and underlying cause, as this has significant implications for treatment and management. Early diagnosis of dementia is crucial

for effective management and treatment planning. It allows for timely interventions that can enhance the quality of life for the affected individual and their family, and it provides an opportunity for planning future care needs. The collaboration between healthcare providers, patients, and families is vital to the diagnostic process and the ongoing care that follows.

Treatment Options for Dementia

While dementia casts a long shadow, with no permanent cure yet discovered, there's solace in knowing it's not an insurmountable challenge. A diverse arsenal of treatment options exists, empowering us to manage symptoms, elevate quality of life, and even potentially slow the disease's relentless march. As the global burden of dementia intensifies, researchers and healthcare professionals remain undeterred, relentlessly pursuing innovative therapies and approaches to illuminate a brighter future.

Let's explore the current landscape of dementia treatment, discovering established practices and the exciting frontiers of ongoing innovation. Here's an in-depth look at the current practices and innovations in memory loss and dementia treatment.

Pharmacological Treatments

Pharmacological treatment for memory loss and dementia constitutes a pivotal aspect of the comprehensive approach to managing cognitive impairments associated with conditions like Alzheimer's disease. As the prevalence of these neurodegenerative disorders continues to rise, pharmaceutical interventions play a central role in alleviating symptoms, enhancing cognitive function, and improving the overall quality of life for affected individuals.

There are a number of pharmacological treatments that can help manage symptoms and improve quality of life. These treatments work by targeting different aspects of the disease process, such as reducing the buildup of harmful proteins in the brain, protecting nerve cells, and improving communication between nerve cells.

Pharmacological treatments for memory loss and dementia can be a valuable tool in helping people live with these conditions.

However, it is important to remember that these treatments are not a cure yet and should be used in conjunction with other lifestyle and support measures. Please talk to your doctor about the treatment options that may be right for you.

Cholinesterase Inhibitors

Cholinesterase inhibitors emerge as a beacon of hope for individuals grappling with mild to moderate Alzheimer's disease, constituting a noteworthy category of medications that actively contribute to managing cognitive decline. By specifically targeting the cholinergic system—a component of the nervous system that plays a role in various physiological functions (cognition, memory, and muscle control), these medications, including Donepezil, Rivastigmine, and Galantamine, play a pivotal role in elevating acetylcholine levels—an essential neurotransmitter for memory and learning. While they don't provide a definitive cure, cholinesterase inhibitors showcase promise in slowing down memory loss and cognitive decline.

Beyond their impact on disease progression, these medications offer a ray of hope by temporarily alleviating cognitive symptoms, ultimately striving to maintain cognitive function and enhance the overall quality of life for both patients and caregivers. Positive outcomes, such as improved memory, enhanced cognitive function, and increased overall cognitive abilities, have been witnessed in some patients.

In essence, cholinesterase inhibitors stand as a vital component in the pharmacological toolkit against Alzheimer's disease, significantly contributing to improved cognitive function and symptom alleviation, offering valuable support for individuals navigating this challenging condition.

NMDA-receptor Antagonists

Imagine your brain as a bustling city, with information constantly zipping along highways called synapses. NMDA receptors act like toll booths, meticulously controlling the flow of information essential for learning and memory. But in dementia, these booths sometimes get stuck open, causing an information overload like a massive traffic jam.

This "overexcitement" damages brain cells and worsens memory loss. This is where NMDA-receptor antagonists step in. Think of them as traffic-calming measures for the brain. They gently nudge the closed toll booths, reducing the overwhelming information flow and protecting brain cells from the damaging effects of overload. This approach holds promise for dementia patients in several ways. Firstly, by quieting the overstimulation, they could potentially slow down memory decline. Secondly, protecting brain cells from overload. With NMDA-receptor antagonists acting as shields, brain health, and memory function might be preserved for longer.

However, it's important to remember that NMDA-receptor antagonists are still under investigation and are not a cure for dementia. They may not work for everyone, and each person responds differently. While these "traffic calming measures" are just one piece of the puzzle, research in this area is exciting. By understanding and fine-tuning how NMDA receptors work, we can hope to unlock even more promising solutions for protecting memory and brain health in the future.

Monoclonal Antibodies

Monoclonal antibodies (mAbs) stand as revolutionary "smart molecules" in the battle against memory loss and dementia, acting as specialized clean-up crews in the intricate landscape of the brain. Engineered to precisely target and eliminate aberrant proteins like beta-amyloid plaques, these mAbs serve as essential components to clear the neural pathways, restoring the smooth flow of information vital for cognitive function. Picture them as vigilant custodians, meticulously removing obstacles that hinder memory and cognition.

Recent strides in mAb development, exemplified by drugs such as lecanemab and aducanumab receiving US approval, mark a pivotal moment in Alzheimer's treatment.

These medications exhibit promising outcomes, showcasing their potential to slow cognitive decline and instill hope for those grappling with this challenging disease. Gantenerumab, another mAb in the spotlight, adds to the excitement with early research suggesting both effectiveness and safety, further validating the promise of this innovative therapeutic approach.

It's important to acknowledge that mAbs are still undergoing investigation, and their efficacy may vary among individuals, accompanied by potential side effects. Nevertheless, the encouraging risk-benefit assessment, with the prospect of slowing cognitive decline, positions mAbs as valuable candidates in the treatment arsenal.

Ongoing research aims to refine and enhance these "clean-up crews," offering a glimpse into a future with even more potent strategies. While the battle against Alzheimer's persists, the emergence of mAbs illuminates a beacon of hope for the millions impacted by this formidable disease.

Lecanemab-irmb, Aducanumab, and Gantenerumab

Lecanemab-irmb, aducanumab, and gantenerumab are anti-amyloid antibodies that have gained attention for their potential in treating Alzheimer's disease. Anti-amyloid antibodies are a class of therapeutic agents designed to target and neutralize amyloid-beta (Aβ) proteins in the brain.

Amyloid-beta is a peptide that accumulates in the brains of individuals with Alzheimer's disease, forming plaques that are associated with neurodegeneration and cognitive decline. These antibodies are part of a class of medications developed to address the underlying pathology of Alzheimer's by binding to and promoting the clearance of amyloid plaques.

Prominent examples of anti-amyloid antibodies include lecanemab-irmb, which has been the subject of research and clinical trials exploring their efficacy in treating Alzheimer's and modifying the disease course. The hope is that these antibodies can provide a targeted approach to addressing the underlying causes of Alzheimer's, offering potential benefits in terms of cognitive preservation and overall disease management.

In a groundbreaking 18-month study, lecanemab exhibited a remarkable 27% reduction in the rate of cognitive decline, marking a significant leap forward in combating Alzheimer's. Collaborative efforts between Eisai and Biogen have presented compelling data for LEQEMBI® (lecanemab-irmb), underscoring its transformative potential. The results showcased clinical improvement and the absence of deterioration in a substantial percentage of the low-tau subpopulation after 18 months of treatment. Results indicated clinical improvement and no deterioration in a considerable percentage after 18 months of treatment.

The ongoing research continues to contribute valuable insights into its effectiveness and safety in treating Alzheimer's disease. In essence, lecanemab-irmb emerges as a promising therapeutic intervention, demonstrating a potential to alter the course of cognitive decline in Alzheimer's patients.

Memantine

Memantine is a valuable treatment option for individuals grappling with moderate to severe Alzheimer's disease. Unlike other Alzheimer's medications aiming to boost neurotransmitter levels, Memantine focuses on regulating glutamate neurotransmitters, the primary excitatory neurotransmitter in the central nervous system. However, excess amounts can lead to overstimulation of nerve cells, resulting in cellular damage and cognitive decline.

What sets Memantine apart is its ability to selectively block NMDA receptors, which are a specific subtype of glutamate receptors. By doing this, Memantine ensures that the signaling pathways remain active but not overly so, essentially protecting the brain cells from the toxic effects of excessive glutamate activity.

The medication acts as a safeguard, helping to maintain the integrity of neural circuits critical for memory and cognition. While Memantine isn't a cure for Alzheimer's, it can be a valuable component of a comprehensive treatment plan. When used with other therapies and medications, it can decelerate the rate of cognitive decline, allowing patients to maintain a better quality of life for a more extended period. Therefore, it often represents a meaningful therapeutic option for patients and healthcare providers dealing with Alzheimer's.

Antipsychotic Medications

Antipsychotic medications are primarily prescribed for managing behavioral and psychological symptoms associated with dementia rather than directly targeting memory loss. These symptoms, collectively known as Behavioral and Psychological Symptoms of Dementia (BPSD), include agitation, aggression, hallucinations, and delusions.

While antipsychotics may help control challenging behaviors in some cases, their use in dementia is not without controversy. Research suggests that conventional antipsychotics may be associated with increased mortality in dementia patients, and atypical antipsychotics, while commonly prescribed, may have limited efficacy.

It's essential to note that antipsychotic medications are not considered a first-line treatment for cognitive symptoms or memory loss in dementia. Other drugs, such as acetylcholinesterase inhibitors like donepezil, are more commonly used to address cognitive decline in conditions like Alzheimer's disease.

Antipsychotic medications are primarily employed for managing behavioral symptoms in dementia, with their use in addressing memory loss being secondary and often associated with potential risks.

Symptomatic Treatments

Symptomatic treatments for memory loss and dementia encompass a range of pharmaceutical interventions designed to alleviate cognitive symptoms associated with conditions like Alzheimer's disease. FDA-approved drugs, including memantine (Namenda) and donepezil (Aricept), are commonly prescribed to manage moderate-to-severe Alzheimer's disease. These medications work by regulating neurotransmitters in the brain, providing relief from memory loss, cognitive decline, and functional impairment.

Additionally, cholinesterase inhibitors, such as rivastigmine and galantamine, form part of the therapeutic arsenal, aiming to enhance acetylcholine levels and mitigate cognitive decline. Selective serotonin reuptake inhibitors (SSRIs) are often utilized for mood symptoms in dementia, contributing to an improved quality of life for individuals affected by these conditions. These interventions, backed by clinical studies and medical guidelines, play an essential role in managing symptoms and improving the daily lives of those affected by memory loss and dementia.

Other medications might be used to treat symptoms associated with dementia, such as depression or sleep disturbances. Still, again, they do not cure the underlying condition. Researchers continue to explore new treatments, including immunotherapies and other targeted therapies, to understand and potentially modify the underlying disease process.

Clinical trials are ongoing, and new medications may be on the horizon. However, as of the last update, no medications can cure dementia. The current focus is typically on symptom management, supporting quality of life, and providing comprehensive care to individuals with dementia and their caregivers.

Combination Therapy

Combination therapy for dementia involves the concurrent use of multiple therapeutic agents to address various aspects of the condition. One notable combination is the use of donepezil and memantine. This fixed-dose combination has demonstrated effectiveness in managing dementia symptoms, providing a comprehensive approach to target different pathways involved in the disease.

Research explores treatment combinations that target multiple disease pathways, such as addressing both amyloid and inflammation in Alzheimer's disease. The choice between monotherapy and combination therapy is an area of discussion.

Studies evaluate the comparative effectiveness of these approaches in managing Alzheimer's disease, contributing to a better understanding of the optimal treatment strategies.

Ongoing initiatives like Alzheimer's Combination Therapy Opportunities (ACTO) focus on identifying promising combination therapies and fostering advancements in the field to enhance treatment outcomes for dementia.

Behavioral and Psychological Therapies

Non-pharmacological therapies have gained traction as an important aspect of holistic dementia care. These therapies aim to manage behavioral and psychological symptoms such as agitation, depression, and anxiety without relying solely on medication. Behavioral and psychological therapies play a fundamental role in enhancing the well-being and quality of life for individuals with dementia. These therapies encompass various approaches tailored to address cognitive and emotional aspects. Some notable therapies include:

Cognitive Behavioral Therapy (CBT)

Cognitive Behavioral Therapy (CBT) in dementia care integrates cognitive and behavioral techniques to address anxiety and behavioral issues. This approach fosters positive coping strategies, empowering patients to navigate challenges associated with their cognitive decline. CBT is designed to enhance emotional resilience and improve adaptive behaviors, contributing to a more positive and supportive care environment.

Occupational Therapy (OT)

Occupational Therapy (OT) focuses on enriching daily life skills to help individuals with dementia maintain independence. Beyond traditional activities, OT includes innovative interventions like reminiscence therapy, music therapy, and cognitive-based activities. These interventions not only promote engagement but also enhance functional abilities, empowering individuals to participate actively in meaningful daily tasks.

Reminiscence Therapy

Reminiscence Therapy encourages individuals to recall and share past experiences, fostering a deep sense of identity and connection. By tapping into personal memories, this therapeutic approach enhances emotional well-being, stimulates cognitive function, and promotes social interaction. Reminiscence therapy creates a bridge between the past and present, contributing to a more enriched and fulfilling life for individuals with dementia.

Problem-Solving Therapy

Led by clinical psychologists, Problem-Solving Therapy is an individualized approach aiming to reduce depression by helping patients identify and tackle specific problems. This therapy equips individuals with practical problem-solving skills, enabling them to navigate challenges effectively and maintain a positive outlook.

Talk Therapy

Effective in the early to middle stages of dementia, talk therapy involves psychological or talking therapies that focus on communication and emotional expression. Facilitating open communication, talk therapy helps individuals express their feelings, fears, and concerns, providing emotional support and enhancing their sense of agency.

Cognitive Stimulation Therapy

Aimed at those with mild to moderate dementia, Cognitive Stimulation Therapy involves engaging in activities specifically designed to stimulate cognitive function. This therapy fosters mental agility, memory recall, and social interaction, contributing to the maintenance of cognitive abilities and overall cognitive well-being.

Reality Orientation Training

Reality Orientation Training is a structured intervention that helps individuals with dementia maintain awareness of time, place, and person. By providing orientation cues and reinforcing a sense of reality, this therapy reduces disorientation, enhances a person's connection to their environment, and promotes a more stable and secure mental state.

Music Therapy (MT)

Music Therapy (MT) utilizes the power of music to stimulate cognitive function, evoke emotions, and enhance social interactions. Tailored to individual preferences, this therapy contributes to memory recall, emotional expression, and overall well-being. Music therapy is known to have a profound impact on individuals with dementia, providing a means of connection and expression when verbal communication becomes challenging.

Stimulation-Oriented Approaches

Stimulation-oriented approaches encompass a spectrum of activities and recreational therapies, including crafts, games, and pet interaction, as well as art therapies like music and dance. These interventions are designed to engage individuals cognitively, emotionally, and socially, providing holistic stimulation that contributes to overall well-being.

These interventions are designed to address the unique challenges associated with dementia, providing therapeutic support to enhance the quality of life for individuals and their caregivers. These therapies aim to enhance cognitive abilities, alleviate behavioral symptoms, and provide emotional support. It's essential to tailor interventions to the individual's specific needs, considering the varying stages and manifestations of dementia.

Lifestyle Modifications

As our understanding of cognitive health advances, it becomes increasingly evident that proactive measures play a pivotal role in maintaining and promoting cognitive well-being. Beyond medical interventions, lifestyle modifications emerge as powerful tools in shaping the trajectory of cognitive aging. These practical strategies will empower you to take charge of your cognitive well-being and navigate the path toward a fulfilling and mentally resilient life:

- *Physical Activity:* Regular exercise, with a recommended minimum of 5 hours per week, correlates with a lower risk of Alzheimer's and vascular dementia. Exercise enhances blood flow to the brain, promoting overall cognitive health and reducing the risk of cognitive decline.

- *Nutrition and Vitamins:* Adopting heart-healthy diets like DASH or the Mediterranean diet, along with sufficient intake of vitamins D, B-complex, and C, has shown potential in lowering the risk of Alzheimer's disease and supporting cognitive health.

- *Adequate Sleep:* Ensuring 7-9 hours of sleep for adults is essential for cognitive health. During this period, the brain clears out beta-amyloid, a substance associated with Alzheimer's disease. Monitoring sleep quality and addressing sleep-related issues are essential considerations.

- *Stress Management:* Chronic stress contributes to various health issues, including cognitive decline.

236

Techniques like yoga, meditation, and mindfulness effectively manage stress, promoting overall well-being and cognitive health.

- **Social Connections:** Maintaining strong social ties and engaging in regular social activities may reduce the risk of cognitive decline and Alzheimer's. Positive social interactions contribute to cognitive benefits, though the exact mechanisms are not fully understood.
- **Avoiding Traumatic Brain Injury (TBI):** Preventing repetitive head trauma, often associated with certain sports or military service, is Important for avoiding Traumatic Brain Injury (TBI). TBI has been linked to an increased risk of dementia later in life, emphasizing the importance of injury prevention for cognitive health.
- **Cognitive Challenges:** Continuously challenging the mind with diverse cognitive exercises, such as crosswords, chess, or learning a new language, can provide additional stimulation. These challenges go beyond routine activities, promoting neuroplasticity and maintaining cognitive flexibility.
- **Hydration:** Proper hydration is essential for overall health, including cognitive function. Dehydration can impair concentration and attention, emphasizing the importance of an adequate daily water intake.
- **Regular Health Check-ups:** Scheduled health check-ups can help identify and address potential health issues early on. Conditions like hypertension and diabetes, when managed effectively, contribute to the overall well-being of the brain.
- **Cognitive Training Programs:** Participating in structured cognitive training programs designed to enhance memory, attention, and problem-solving skills can be beneficial. These programs are tailored to stimulate specific cognitive functions and may offer protective effects against cognitive decline.
- **Mindful Screen Time:** Balancing screen time and incorporating mindful practices while using electronic devices can contribute to mental well-being. Excessive screen time, especially on social media, may impact mental health negatively.
- **Continued Learning:** Embracing a mindset of lifelong learning encourages intellectual curiosity. Pursuing new

interests or taking courses stimulates the brain, contributing to cognitive reserve and resilience against cognitive decline.

- **Moderation in Alcohol Consumption:** While moderate alcohol consumption may have some cardiovascular benefits, excessive alcohol intake can harm cognitive function. Maintaining moderation aligns with overall brain health.
- **Environmental Enrichment:** Creating an enriched living environment with stimulating elements like art, music, or nature can positively impact cognitive health. An enriched environment fosters sensory experiences that benefit brain function.
- **Smoking Cessation:** Quitting smoking or avoiding it altogether is essential to reduce the risks of heart disease and stroke, both contributing factors to an increased likelihood of developing dementia.

From mentally stimulating activities to the importance of sleep, nutrition, and social connections, each aspect contributes to a holistic approach aimed at safeguarding the intricate workings of the human brain. By adopting these lifestyle modifications, you can not only potentially delay the onset of cognitive decline but also enhance their overall quality of life.

Antioxidants and Nutritional Supplements

Oxidative stress, characterized by an imbalance between free radicals and antioxidants in the body, has been implicated in the development of memory loss and various neurodegenerative diseases. The brain, being highly susceptible to oxidative damage due to its high metabolic activity and lipid-rich composition, faces increased vulnerability to free radical attacks. In response to this, researchers have investigated the potential benefits of antioxidant supplements in mitigating oxidative stress and preserving cognitive function.

Vitamins E and C, renowned for their antioxidant properties, have been subjects of extensive investigation. Vitamin E, with its lipid-soluble nature, may protect cell membranes from oxidative damage, while Vitamin C's water-soluble nature allows it to neutralize free radicals in the aqueous environment of cells. Additionally, omega-3 fatty acids, found in abundance in fatty fish, have shown promise in supporting brain health by reducing inflammation and oxidative stress.

However, the outcomes of studies exploring the efficacy of antioxidant supplements in preventing memory loss and neurodegenerative diseases have been variable. While some trials suggest potential neuroprotective effects, others present inconclusive results. As a more holistic approach, adopting a well-balanced diet rich in antioxidants and essential nutrients appears to be a prudent strategy. This dietary approach not only provides a spectrum of antioxidants but also ensures a synergistic effect, as various nutrients work in tandem to support overall brain health. Incorporating colorful fruits and vegetables, nuts, seeds, and fatty fish into one's diet can contribute to the multifaceted protection against oxidative stress, potentially positively impacting both memory and the overall well-being of the brain.

Emerging Therapies

As cognitive research expands, novel treatments begin to enter the arena. Although more recently developed, many of these emerging therapies have undergone rigorous testing to prove efficacy and safety. Some of these therapies are still undergoing testing. To promote your health and advance the knowledge of these treatments for the public, you may choose to enroll as a participant in a clinical trial. To determine your eligibility and the costs and benefits of participating in a clinical trial, speak to your healthcare provider. Here are some of the more recent developments in the cognitive science community:

Immunotherapy

Recent strides in immunotherapy present a hopeful avenue for addressing Alzheimer's disease by targeting a key pathology—amyloid plaques. Amyloid plaques, composed of abnormal clumps of protein, are implicated in the neurodegenerative process leading to memory loss in Alzheimer's patients. Monoclonal antibodies, exemplified by aducanumab, have emerged as a forefront strategy aiming to clear these plaques from the brain.

Aducanumab, a monoclonal antibody of the IgG1 class, demonstrates a targeted approach directed at amyloid beta, a major component of these plaques. The therapeutic goal is to facilitate the removal of amyloid plaques, potentially halting or slowing the progression of memory loss associated with Alzheimer's disease. This approach signifies a shift from conventional symptomatic treatments to a more disease-modifying strategy.

While these immunotherapeutic interventions offer promise, the long-term effectiveness and potential side effects necessitate further investigation. Ongoing research, including clinical trials and real-world studies, aims to comprehensively understand the safety and efficacy profiles of these monoclonal antibodies.

The hope is that these advancements will contribute significantly to reshaping Alzheimer's disease therapeutics, offering not just symptomatic relief but potentially altering the course of the disease itself.

Gene Therapies

As the understanding of genetic factors influencing memory loss and cognitive decline advances, gene therapies are emerging as a promising frontier in Alzheimer's disease research. Scientists are actively exploring innovative approaches to target and modify specific genes associated with neurodegeneration, aiming to enhance brain function and safeguard neurons.

Recent human gene therapy trials for Alzheimer's disease have showcased encouraging results in preclinical studies, demonstrating the potential of this novel treatment avenue. The primary goal is to deliver healthy genes or modulate existing ones, addressing the underlying genetic components that contribute to cognitive decline. In some instances, researchers are investigating gene silencing strategies to mitigate the impact of genes associated with Alzheimer's.

For instance, ongoing clinical trials are assessing the safety and efficacy of gene therapies in Alzheimer's patients. These trials aim to evaluate the feasibility of this approach, exploring its potential to not only halt cognitive decline but also promote cognitive function restoration.

While gene therapies for Alzheimer's are still in the early stages of development, the progress made in preclinical and clinical studies provides hope for a future where targeted genetic interventions could revolutionize the treatment landscape for memory-related disorders.

Stem Cell Therapy

Stem cell therapy presents a compelling avenue for regenerating damaged brain tissue and fostering neuroplasticity. Preliminary studies on animal models have demonstrated encouraging outcomes, showcasing the potential of stem cells in promoting neural repair and recovery. These versatile cells hold the promise of differentiating into various cell types, contributing to tissue regeneration and functional improvement.

In preclinical trials, researchers have observed positive effects such as enhanced neurotrophic factor secretion, improved axon regeneration, and reduced astrogliosis after traumatic brain injury. These findings suggest that stem cells, when integrated with biological scaffolds, can be implanted into damaged areas to facilitate the repair process.

Despite these promising developments, significant challenges persist in translating these preclinical successes into safe and effective treatments for humans. The complexity of the human brain, ethical considerations, and the need for rigorous clinical testing pose hurdles that researchers must overcome to ensure the viability and safety of stem cell therapy in treating brain-related conditions.

Ongoing research endeavors aim to address these challenges and unlock the full therapeutic potential of stem cell therapy for brain regeneration. As scientists continue to unravel the intricacies of stem cell behavior and refine their techniques, the future holds promise for innovative treatments that harness the power of stem cells to heal and rejuvenate the human brain.

Cognitive Training Programs

In the realm of cognitive enhancement, computer-based cognitive training programs have emerged as promising tools harnessing technological advancements. These programs are meticulously designed to address and enhance specific cognitive functions, notably targeting memory and attention. The primary objective is to improve overall cognitive abilities, offering potential benefits for individuals experiencing memory loss or cognitive decline.

Several studies have explored the efficacy of these programs. A pilot randomized, controlled trial investigated intensive, computer-based cognitive training in subjects with mild cognitive impairment, demonstrating its potential in addressing cognitive challenges. Another clinical trial implemented a 45-minute cognitive training session twice a week, highlighting the impact of computer-based cognitive training on cognitive functions.

The programs often incorporate guided drills and practices tailored to single or multiple cognitive domains. This approach aims to provide a comprehensive and targeted intervention for individuals seeking cognitive improvement. Moreover, the advent of personalized online brain training, such as CogniFit's, a cognitive training program intended to help users improve brain functioning, emphasizes the individualized stimulation, training, and rehabilitation of key cognitive skills.

While these computer-based cognitive training programs show promise in enhancing cognitive abilities, ongoing research is vital to fully understand their long-term effectiveness and potential implications for memory loss and cognitive disorders.

Virtual Reality (VR) and Augmented Reality (AR)

Virtual Reality (VR) and Augmented Reality (AR) have emerged as innovative tools in the realm of cognitive training and memory rehabilitation. These immersive technologies offer the potential to enhance cognitive abilities by simulating real-life scenarios and providing engaging experiences.

Research indicates that VR and AR interventions can lead to improvements in various cognitive domains, including memory, dual-tasking, processing, and attention. Cognitive-motor interventions based on VR have demonstrated moderate to large effects on global cognition, attention, memory, and motor skills. Furthermore, these technologies are explored for the rehabilitation of acquired cognitive impairments, showing promise in assisting individuals with neurological conditions.

Fully immersive VR has been investigated as a useful intervention in cognitive rehabilitation across different conditions. The potential of immersive VR for cognitive assessment and training is recognized, allowing for the measurement of subtle cognitive changes in diagnostic and rehabilitation settings. These technologies can be categorized into three main applications: stimulation, training, and cognitive rehabilitation, each contributing to the development of tailored interventions.

While the field is evolving, the integration of VR and AR in cognitive training holds great promise for creating personalized and effective interventions to stimulate memory recall and improve overall cognitive function.

Neurofeedback

Neurofeedback, a biofeedback technique, empowers individuals to monitor and regulate their brain activity. The method holds promise in enhancing memory by training individuals to modulate specific brainwaves associated with memory processes. Research suggests that neurofeedback training can effectively improve both episodic and semantic memory. Additionally, studies demonstrate its ability to enhance attention, working memory performance, and theta activity in the resting state.

The benefits of neurofeedback for memory improvement include its potential for long-lasting effects. By addressing the root of memory-related issues and effectively rewiring the brain, neurofeedback offers a holistic approach to memory enhancement. Moreover, findings indicate that neurofeedback may benefit individuals with mild cognitive impairment, suggesting improved memory performance that could be maintained beyond the training period.

Neurofeedback emerges as a promising avenue for memory enhancement, providing individuals with a personalized and targeted approach to optimize their cognitive functions.

Pharmacological Interventions

Recent developments in brain health and aging research showcase promising interventions to prevent, identify, and manage cognitive decline. Researchers are uncovering new roles for proteins that play key roles in memory, with potential implications for enhancing memory and alleviating negative memories associated with conditions like PTSD. A groundbreaking study has identified a novel treatment that reverses signs of Alzheimer's disease, demonstrating improvements in sleep quality, cognitive test performance, and the normalization of proteostasis (the dynamic process by which cells maintain the proper folding, function, and levels of proteins) in mice.

Scientific rigor is being applied to the investigation of herbal supplements purported to improve memory, aiming to provide botanical treatments for memory loss and more effective supplements. Additionally, insights into the nature of memory are emerging, revealing cellular-level mechanisms that could contribute to advancing our understanding and potentially improving memory function.

Brain-Computer Interfaces (BCIs)

Brain-computer interfaces (BCIs) represent innovative systems designed to establish direct communication between the brain and external devices. These interfaces hold immense potential for memory restoration by enabling the facilitation of memory recall through neural pathways. BCIs operate by decoding neural signals, allowing individuals to interact with computers or other devices solely through their thoughts.

This groundbreaking technology opens up possibilities for restoring and enhancing cognitive functions, including memory, by establishing a direct link between the brain and external systems. As advancements in BCI research continue, the potential applications for memory-related interventions and improvements are a promising avenue for the future.

Artificial Intelligence (AI)

AI technologies are being integrated into memory-assistance devices and apps to provide personalized cognitive training and memory support. AI assistive technologies have expanded significantly in recent years, providing a wide array of solutions to improve the quality of life for people with dementia and their caregivers. Below are some ways technology is utilized in this context:

- **Reminder Systems:** One of the simplest forms of assistive technology, reminder systems can benefit someone struggling with memory loss. Digital calendars, smartphone apps, or even specialized devices can be programmed to send alerts for medication times, appointments, and other important events.

- **GPS Tracking:** Wandering can be a significant concern for caregivers of dementia patients. GPS-enabled devices, often wearable like a watch or a pendant, allow caregivers to track the movements of their loved ones. Geo-fencing features can send alerts if the individual leaves a predefined safe area.

- **Smart Home Systems:** Devices like smart lights, thermostats, and door locks can be programmed to adapt to the routines of individuals with dementia. For instance, lights can be set to turn on or off based on time or activity, providing both safety and convenience.

- **Communication Aids:** Tablets and smartphones can be customized with large, easy-to-read interfaces to help people with dementia communicate more effectively. Video calling apps can also enable better connection with friends and family, which can be critical for emotional well-being.

- **Cognitive Training Apps:** These apps are designed to provide mental stimulation through games and exercises that target various cognitive skills like memory, problem-solving, and attention. While they are not a cure for dementia, they can be a part of an overall strategy to maintain cognitive function.

- **AI-Driven Solutions:** Advanced AI technologies, including machine learning algorithms, can analyze behavioral and physiological data to detect patterns or changes in the condition of someone with dementia. This can provide caregivers and medical professionals with valuable insights into treatment and intervention strategies.
- **Robotics:** Robots equipped with AI capabilities can serve multiple roles, from companionship to assistance with daily tasks. They can be programmed to remind patients to take medications, alert caregivers in emergencies, and provide social interaction, reducing feelings of isolation.

Psychedelics

Psychedelic research is experiencing a renaissance after decades of being largely dormant. This renewed interest is due in part to the promising results of early studies into the potential of psychedelics to treat a variety of mental health conditions, including anxiety, depression, and addiction. More recently, researchers have begun to explore the potential of psychedelics to treat memory loss and dementia.

New research shows how psychedelics improve memory and cognition. Classic psychedelics such as Lysergic acid diethylamide (LSD) and psilocybin (the active ingredient in magic mushrooms) can impair some types of memory tasks, such as those that require recalling specific details. Still, they can also enhance other kinds of memory, such as those that rely on familiarity. Psychedelics can increase the vividness and recall of autobiographical memories, which may have therapeutic implications for mental health disorders.

Psychedelics can also increase cognitive flexibility and creativity by reducing the rigidity of prior beliefs and enhancing the generation of novel associations. The latest studies use a neurocognitive model that links the acute and persisting effects of psychedelics on cognition with their therapeutic potential.

Some studies have also explored the possible benefits of psychedelics for Alzheimer's disease. Psychedelics may promote neuroplasticity, the ability of the brain to form new connections and adapt to changes. Neuroplasticity is impaired in Alzheimer's disease, and psychedelics may help restore it by stimulating the growth of new brain cells and synapses.

The potential of psychedelics for Alzheimer's research mentions some ongoing clinical trials that are testing the effects of psilocybin and LSD on cognitive function, mood, and quality of life in patients with mild to moderate Alzheimer's disease. Challenges and limitations include ethical issues, safety concerns, and regulatory barriers.

While the research on psychedelics and memory loss is still in its early stages, the results are promising. More research is needed to confirm these findings and to determine the optimal dosage and treatment regimen for different types of memory loss. However, the potential of psychedelics to treat memory loss is a significant breakthrough in the field of dementia research.

Where to Get Help If You're Concerned About Dementia

If you're concerned that you or someone you know might be exhibiting signs of dementia, taking prompt action is essential. Here are some places where you can seek help and guidance:

- **Primary Care Physician:** Your first port of call should be your general practitioner or primary care physician. They can conduct an initial assessment and perform basic cognitive tests or refer you to specialists for further evaluation.
- **Specialists:** Neurologists, geriatricians, or psychiatrists with expertise in cognitive disorders can provide a more thorough evaluation. They are often better equipped to diagnose and manage dementia and other neurological conditions.
- **Memory Clinics:** These specialized centers focus exclusively on diagnosing and treating memory disorders like dementia. They offer comprehensive assessments and can be a valuable resource for both diagnosis and ongoing care.
- **Support Groups:** Organizations like the Alzheimer's Association offer a range of resources, including support groups for patients and caregivers. These can be valuable for emotional support and practical advice.
- **Online Forums:** Various online platforms offer community support, where you can share experiences, concerns, and advice with people who are going through similar challenges.

- *Social Services:* Government and non-government organizations often provide services like home visits, day-care centers, and respite care for caregivers. Reach out to local agencies to see what assistance may be available.
- *Legal and Financial Planning:* Given the long-term nature of dementia, it's advisable to consult experts for legal and financial planning. This could involve making a will, setting up a power of attorney, and understanding long-term care costs.
- *Pharmacist:* Medication management can become challenging as dementia progresses. A pharmacist can guide medication timing, side effects, and potential interactions.
- *Telehealth Services:* These can provide convenient access to healthcare consultations, particularly for those with mobility issues or who live in remote locations.
- *Psychologists and Counselors:* Emotional and psychological support can be fundamental, especially in the early stages when the individual and their family are coming to terms with the diagnosis.
- *Family and Friends:* Never underestimate the power of a strong support network. Emotional support from loved ones can make a significant difference in the well-being of the person affected by dementia.

If you are concerned about dementia symptoms, seeking professional advice for an accurate diagnosis and appropriate management is essential. These professionals can conduct comprehensive assessments, including medical history reviews, physical examinations, cognitive tests, and sometimes imaging studies, to determine the underlying cause of the symptoms. Everyone's experience with dementia can be different, so tailored care is essential.

Caring for Someone with Dementia

Dementia care is daunting, but it may not be as challenging as one might expect. Whether caring for a parent or senior loved one with Alzheimer's disease or another form of dementia or if you are a senior care professional, approaching the role with some knowledge is Important to the right attitude.

Dementia education and a positive but realistic attitude allow the caregiver to maintain an element of control; this can take the sting out of surprising challenges and enhance care. When approaching the role of caring for someone with dementia, here are some important facts to consider:

Accept Support

Whether caring for someone or providing care professionally, never be afraid to ask for help. Many family caregivers find support groups extremely helpful. Support groups allow caregivers to vent in a group setting with people who understand what each other is going through. It also enables caregivers to hear what is working for other caregivers and learn about local Alzheimer's and dementia resources.

Similarly, professional caregivers should not be reluctant to ask a colleague for support when faced with an unprecedented challenge or a difficult time. Care for someone with dementia is not easy, and there will undoubtedly be times when professional caregivers need a hand or someone to talk to.

Actively Empathize

Care begins with compassion and kindness; this holds true in all human relationships but may be essential for dementia caregivers. People with dementia, for example, are likely to become confused about their whereabouts and even the time they live. For example, imagine how one would want to be treated if suddenly found bewildered in an unfamiliar place, unsure of the year, or even their own identity.

Be a Realistic Caregiver

Be rational in what constitutes success in the progression of the disease. Success helps ensure that the person cared for is as relaxed, satisfied, and healthy as possible. Many seasoned dementia caregivers say the person they care for has good and bad days. Promote good days and even good times for a person with dementia; do not try to push them. It is also essential to be realistic about the course of the disease.

Know that most forms of dementia, including Alzheimer's, are permanent and progressive. Dementia appears to get worse over time, and there is no proven treatment for it. The notable exception is drug-induced dementia, which can be reversed when a medicine is withdrawn.

Dementia is More Than Memory Loss

Memory loss is a typical symptom of dementia. But some forms of dementia, particularly frontotemporal dementia, and Pick's disease, manifest themselves as a change of personality rather than a loss of memory. Symptoms depend on the regions of the brain that are affected by the disease. Even when memory loss is the most apparent symptom, a person with dementia is undergoing a neurological deterioration that can lead to other problems.

A patient can develop challenging behaviors and moods. For example, a fine and proper grandma may begin to curse like a sailor. Or a formally trusting gentleman may believe that his family is conspiring against him or having other visions and hallucinations. At the most recent stage of most forms of dementia, patients cannot engage independently in everyday life tasks (such as dressing and grooming). They can become non-communicative, unable to remember loved ones, and even unable to move about.

Plan for The Future

The only inevitable is 'change' when caring for those with dementia. Never get so used to the status quo; this means that family members should plan for a period when their loved one will require professional memory care in a residential environment. This care includes financial preparation and the selection of the most suitable care choices. Professional caregivers and memory services will need to prepare ahead. They should be aware of constantly reassessing the health and care needs of clients and dementia residents. Note that care needs will eventually increase and prepare ahead for any changes that a resident will need, such as a transfer to a qualified nursing or hospital care provider.

End-of-Life Care

In the later stages of dementia, a compassionate and thoughtful approach to end-of-life care becomes paramount. Prioritizing comfort, preserving dignity, and respecting the wishes of both the individual and their family are central tenets. Managing dementia involves a multifaceted strategy encompassing medical, psychological, lifestyle, and supportive interventions.

Ongoing research continually expands our comprehension of this intricate disorder, opening avenues for innovative treatments that hold promise for enhanced outcomes. Successful dementia care hinges on a patient-centered approach, considering the specific type and stage of dementia alongside the unique needs and preferences of the individual and their family.

The collaborative efforts of healthcare professionals, caregivers, and community resources are indispensable in delivering comprehensive and compassionate care. This collaborative approach aims to enhance the quality of life for individuals navigating the challenges of dementia. As we advance our understanding and treatment options through research, the ultimate goal remains to provide dignified and person-centered care for those with dementia and their families.

Resources for People Living with Dementia

The following list of resources has been selected to help patients and families learn more about dementia, cope with the disease together, and live the best life possible.

- **Alzheimer's Association (www.alz.org)**
  Formed in 1980, the Alzheimer's Association is the leading voluntary health organization in Alzheimer's care, support, and research.

- **National Institute on Aging (www.nia.nih.gov)**
  The National Institute on Aging (NIA), one of the 27 Institutes and Centers of the National Institutes of Health (NIH), leads a broad scientific effort to understand the nature of aging and to extend the healthy, active years of life. NIA is the primary Federal agency supporting and conducting Alzheimer's disease research.

- **Alzheimer's Foundation of America (www.alzfdn.org)**
  The Alzheimer's Foundation of America's (AFA) mission is to provide optimal care and services to individuals living with Alzheimer's disease and related illnesses and to their families and caregivers.

Resources for Caregivers

The following list of resources has been selected to help you learn more about dementia, how to care for your body and mind, and how to provide the best care possible.

- **Alzheimer's Association (www.alz.org)**
  Formed in 1980, the Alzheimer's Association is the leading voluntary health organization in Alzheimer's care, support, and research.

- **National Institute on Aging (www.nia.nih.gov)**
  The National Institute on Aging (NIA), one of the 27 Institutes and Centers of the National Institutes of Health (NIH), leads a broad scientific effort to understand the nature of aging and to extend the healthy, active years of life. NIA is the primary Federal agency supporting and conducting Alzheimer's disease research.

- **Alzheimer's Foundation of America (www.alzfdn.org)**
  The Alzheimer's Foundation of America's (AFA) mission is to provide optimal care and services to individuals living with Alzheimer's disease and related illnesses and to their families and caregivers.

- **AARP (www.aarp.org/caregiving)**
  AARP is a nonprofit, nonpartisan organization that empowers people to choose how they live as they age.

- **Family Caregiver Alliance® (www.caregiver.org)**
  Family Caregiver Alliance is the first community-based nonprofit organization in the country to address the needs of families and friends providing long-term care for loved ones at home.

- **Eldercare Locator (www.eldercare.acl.gov)**
  A public service of the U.S. Administration on Aging connects you to services for older adults and their families.

- **Personal Emergency Response System (PERS)**
  1-877-382-4357
  (TTY: 1-866-653-4261)

Reflections on Navigating Dementia's Challenges

Navigating the challenges of dementia is an emotional and complex journey that requires resilience, empathy, and a deep understanding of the evolving landscape. It's like embarking on an unpredictable voyage where each day unfolds as a unique chapter, bringing triumphs and tribulations.

Imagine a world together in an extraordinary alliance to face one of humanity's most mysterious and heart-wrenching challenges:

dementia. From the corridors of power in government buildings to community halls and individual households to global health organizations, people are rallying around a shared mission. This isn't just about policy changes or medical breakthroughs; it's a crusade powered by the heartbeat of human connection.

Picture awareness campaigns that do more than inform; they shatter taboos and build bridges of understanding. Visualize international pacts that aren't just signatures on paper but are life-changing collaborations with no borders. We're talking about a genuine, world-spanning commitment to uplift those with dementia and provide solace to their families.

Feel the emotional undercurrent in the stories that bubble up from this movement—the tender tales of caregivers, the deeply personal experiences of families, and the inspiring accounts from those bravely navigating life with dementia. These narratives echo in our hearts and minds, reminding us that amid the struggle and complexity of dementia, our capacity for love, empathy, and compassion remains unbreakable.

Yes, dementia is an imposing mountain to climb. Still, humanity is taking on the ascent with ropes tied together by determination and hope. This isn't just a healthcare quest; it's a soulful journey that taps into the core of our shared human spirit. We're recognizing that each person grappling with dementia is more than a diagnosis; they're carriers of unique stories, keepers of invaluable legacies, and important members of our global community.

So, what's on the horizon? Picture a landscape ripe with innovation, teeming with scientific curiosity, and enriched by cultural understanding. Imagine a future where dignity in dementia care is a given, not an exception. We're not just aspiring to manage this condition but actively working to defeat it. The beacon of hope in this endeavor isn't merely flickering; it's a blazing torch that lights up the path for all of us, inviting everyone to be an active, compassionate, and hopeful player in the noble struggle against dementia.

The time is now, and the road ahead is ours to travel. Let's make it a journey of hope, unity, and relentless human spirit. Join the fight; be part of this incredible global movement. Because together, we're not just powerful; we're unstoppable.

Glossary

A

Adaptation: The process of adjusting to new information and experiences. It involves modifying behaviors, attitudes, or responses to fit changing circumstances better and improve overall functioning.

Aerobic Exercise: Physical activity that increases heart rate and promotes cardiovascular health. Examples include running, swimming, and cycling, which enhance oxygen circulation and positively affect overall well-being.

Alzheimer's Disease: A progressive neurological disorder characterized by memory loss, cognitive decline, and behavioral changes. It is the most common cause of dementia, affecting memory, thinking, and the ability to perform daily activities.

Amygdala: A part of the brain located in the temporal lobe, the amygdala processes emotions, particularly fear responses. It also plays a role in memory formation, especially for emotionally charged events.

Anticholinergic Medications: Drugs that block the neurotransmitter acetylcholine in the brain. They are used for various medical purposes but can have side effects, including impairments in memory and cognition.

Antioxidants: Substances that protect cells against damage from free radicals and oxidative stress. They are found in certain foods and are believed to have potential health benefits, including cognitive protection.

Artificial Intelligence (AI): Computer systems capable of performing tasks that typically require human intelligence. AI includes machine learning, natural language processing, and other technologies that simulate human cognitive functions.

Autobiographical Memory: The aspect of memory related to personal experiences and facts about one's life. It includes memories of significant events, emotions, and personal narratives.

B

Brain Plasticity: Also known as neuroplasticity, the brain can change and reorganize over the lifespan by forming new connections between neurons. This process allows the brain to adapt to learning, experience, and recovery from injury.

Brain Stimulation: Techniques for activating or altering brain activity using electricity, magnets, or implants. This includes methods like transcranial magnetic stimulation (TMS) and deep brain stimulation (DBS), used for therapeutic purposes.

Brain-Computer Interfaces (BCIs): Technologies that enable direct communication between the brain and external devices, such as computers. BCIs can be used for various applications, including assisting individuals with paralysis.

Brain-Gut Connection: The bidirectional communication between the brain and the gastrointestinal system. It highlights the impact of gut health on mental well-being and cognitive function.

C

Cognitive Decline: The gradual worsening of cognitive abilities, including memory, attention, and reasoning. It is often associated with aging, but certain conditions, such as dementia, can accelerate cognitive decline.

Cognitive Functions: Mental processes and skills involved in perception, thinking, reasoning, memory, and language. These functions collectively contribute to how individuals process and understand information.

Cognitive Processes: The mental activities involved in acquiring, processing, storing, and using information. These processes include perception, attention, memory, language, problem-solving, and decision-making.

Cognitive Reserve: The brain's ability to function despite age-related changes or damage. Education, intellectual activities, and a stimulating environment contribute to cognitive reserve.

Cognitive Training: Structured practice on tasks related to mental functions like memory, attention, and problem-solving. Cognitive training programs aim to enhance specific cognitive abilities through repetitive exercises.

Confirmation Bias: The tendency to seek and favor information that confirms existing beliefs while ignoring or dismissing contradictory evidence. It can lead to distorted perceptions and reinforce preexisting views.

Concept Mapping and Diagrams: Graphical tools organize and represent relationships between ideas and concepts. They help in visualizing information, making it easier to understand and remember.

Cranial Electrotherapy Stimulation (CES): A therapeutic technique involving the application of a low-voltage electrical current to the brain through electrodes on the earlobes. CES is sometimes used to treat certain mental health conditions.

Cross-Racial Identification Errors: Difficulty accurately recognizing and recalling the faces of individuals from different racial or ethnic backgrounds. It highlights the influence of cultural factors on facial recognition.

Cryptomnesia: A memory bias where individuals believe they generated a new idea that they encountered previously but have forgotten. It can lead to unintentional plagiarism and a false sense of originality.

D

Decision-Making Systems: Parts of the brain involved in evaluating options and selecting appropriate actions. Decision-making systems are crucial in choosing behaviors based on available information and goals.

Deep Brain Stimulation (DBS): A surgical procedure involving the implantation of electrodes in specific brain regions to deliver electrical impulses. DBS is used as a treatment for certain neurological conditions, including Parkinson's disease.

Dementia: A progressive cognitive decline that interferes with daily functioning. Dementia is characterized by memory loss, impaired reasoning, and changes in behavior. Alzheimer's disease is a common cause of dementia.

Digital Hobbies: Leisure activities involving digital technologies, such as computers, video games, or robotics. Engaging in digital hobbies can have both recreational and cognitive benefits.

E

Echoic Memory: Ultra-short-term auditory memory lasting up to 3-4 seconds. Echoic memory allows individuals to temporarily retain and process auditory information, such as sounds and spoken words, for a brief duration.

Electroencephalogram (EEG): A method of recording and analyzing electrical brain activity using electrodes placed on the scalp. EEG is a non-invasive technique that provides insights into brain function and is widely used in clinical and research settings.

End-of-life Care: Medical care and support provided at the end of one's life, either due to age or terminal illness. End-of-care focuses on ensuring comfort and quality of life and addressing individuals' physical, emotional, and spiritual needs.

Episodic Memory: The ability to remember specific events, situations, and experiences in one's life. Episodic memory involves recalling contextual details, such as time, place, and emotions associated with the events.

Episodic Memory Tests: Assessments designed to evaluate a person's ability to recall specific details of experiences and episodes. These tests often involve presenting individuals with scenarios or events and measuring their ability to remember and describe the details.

Executive Function: Cognitive processes that regulate thoughts and behaviors, including planning, organization, focus, and impulse control. Executive function is essential for goal-directed behavior and the successful completion of tasks.

Explicit (Declarative) Memory: Conscious, intentional recollection of facts, events, and concepts. This type of memory involves deliberately retrieving information that can be consciously brought into awareness.

Eyewitness Testimony Errors: Inaccuracies in recalling details when providing eyewitness accounts of crimes or events. Factors such as stress, leading questions, and biases can contribute to errors in eyewitness testimony.

F

False Memories: Recalling events that did not occur or distorting actual memories. False memories can be influenced by suggestion, misinformation, or other cognitive factors, leading individuals to believe in the truth of events that never happened.

Fragmented Memory: Patchy recall of an event where some aspects can be remembered, but other details are missing. Fragmented memory can result from various factors, including trauma or stress, leading to an incomplete recollection of an experience.

G

Galantamine: A medication used to treat Alzheimer's disease by increasing acetylcholine levels in the brain. Acetylcholine is a neurotransmitter involved in memory and learning, and galantamine aims to enhance its activity to mitigate cognitive decline in Alzheimer's patients.

Gene Therapy: The introduction or alteration of genes to treat diseases like Alzheimer's and dementia. In the context of memory-related disorders, gene therapy explores genetic interventions to address underlying causes or factors contributing to cognitive decline.

H

Haptic Memory: Memory involves touch sensations, textures, shapes, and movements. Haptic memory allows individuals to recall and recognize objects or experiences based on their sense of touch.

Hippocampus: Part of the brain is critical for forming new memories and accessing recall. The hippocampus is fundamental in consolidating short-term memories into long-term storage and is essential for spatial navigation and memory recall.

Hormones: Chemical messengers like estrogen, testosterone, and cortisol influence brain function and memory. Hormones play a role in regulating various physiological processes, including those related to mood, stress response, and cognitive function.

Hyperthyroidism: A medical condition characterized by excess thyroid hormone production. Hyperthyroidism can impact cognitive function, including memory, and may lead to symptoms such as difficulty concentrating and memory lapses.

Hypothyroidism: A medical condition characterized by insufficient thyroid hormones. Hypothyroidism can affect cognitive function, leading to symptoms such as memory lapses, sluggishness, and difficulty concentrating. Hormone replacement therapy is often used to manage this condition.

I

Iconic Memory: Brief visual memory store lasting a fraction of a second after seeing something. Iconic memory allows individuals to retain a snapshot of visual information for a very short duration, contributing to the continuity of visual perception.

Imagination Inflation: False memories are formed when imagining counterfactual events. Imagination inflation occurs when vividly imagining events that did not happen can lead to a person believing in the truth of those imagined events.

Immunotherapy: Treatments that harness the immune system to fight diseases like Alzheimer's. Immunotherapy in memory disorders involves using the body's immune system to target and eliminate harmful substances, such as beta-amyloid plaques implicated in Alzheimer's disease.

Implicit (Procedural) Memory: Unconscious memory for skills, habits, primal associations, and reactions. Implicit memory involves the automatic recall of information without conscious effort and is often associated with procedural learning and motor skills.

Impaired Synaptic Function: Disruption in communication between neurons at synapses negatively impacts memory. When the synaptic function is impaired, the transmission of signals between neurons is compromised, affecting cognitive processes, including memory formation and retrieval.

Individual Variability: Natural diversity among individuals in traits like memory capacity. Individual variability recognizes that people differ in their cognitive abilities, including memory, due to genetic, environmental, and experiential factors.

L

Lewy Body Dementia (LBD): Dementia with Lewy bodies (abnormal protein deposits) that affects memory. Lewy body dementia is a progressive neurological disorder characterized by cognitive decline, visual hallucinations, and motor symptoms, with memory impairment being one aspect of the condition.

Life-long Learning: Ongoing acquisition of knowledge and skills throughout the lifespan. Lifelong learning emphasizes the continuous pursuit of education and personal development across one's entire life, promoting cognitive health and adaptability.

Life-long Rehabilitation: Providing therapy and support services continually as a person ages. Lifelong rehabilitation involves ongoing efforts to maintain or improve cognitive and physical functioning throughout an individual's life, which is particularly important in age-related conditions.

Lecanemabirmb (Leqembi): An IV medication for clearing amyloid beta plaques implicated in Alzheimer's disease. Lecanemabirmb is a drug designed to target and clear amyloid beta plaques, a hallmark of Alzheimer's disease, to slow cognitive decline.

Long-Term Memory Tests: Assessments of memory for facts, events, and skills acquired in the distant past. Long-term memory tests evaluate an individual's ability to recall information stored in their memory for an extended period, reflecting the durability of memory.

M

478 Method: A memorization technique that involves associating numbers with consonant sounds. The 478 Method is used as a mnemonic strategy to aid in recalling numerical sequences by converting them into memorable words or phrases.

Memory Assistive Technologies: Devices and apps designed to augment or compensate for memory difficulties. Memory assistive technologies include tools designed to support individuals with memory impairments, such as reminders, organizers, and digital devices.

Memory Care: Specialized assisted living with services tailored to those with dementia and memory loss. Memory care facilities provide a supportive environment for individuals with memory disorders, offering specialized services and programs to enhance their quality of life.

Memory Chunking: Grouping information into smaller meaningful units to aid memorization. Memory chunking is a cognitive strategy that involves breaking down large amounts of data into smaller, manageable chunks to facilitate easier recall.

Memory Chunking and Grouping: Organizing information into related categories or chunks to enhance encoding and recall. This process involves grouping related pieces of information to improve memory organization and retrieval.

Memory Consolidation: Transferring and stabilizing newly learned information from short-term to long-term memory. Memory consolidation is crucial for forming lasting memories and involves strengthening neural connections over time.

Memory Contamination: Errors in recollection due to integrating incorrect external information that distorts the original memory. Memory contamination occurs when inaccurate details are introduced, leading to a distorted recollection of events.

Memory Decay: The fading of memories over time due to disuse, interference, or neurobiological changes. Memory decay reflects the natural process by which memories may become less accessible or vivid over time.

Memory Enhancement: Improving memory encoding, storage, and retrieval through mnemonics. Memory enhancement techniques, such as mnemonics, aim to optimize memory processes and aid in efficiently recalling information.

Memory Problems: Issues with effectively acquiring, retaining, and recalling information. Memory problems can manifest as difficulties in various memory domains, impacting daily functioning and quality of life.

Memory Process: The stages of forming, retaining, and accessing memories. The memory process encompasses encoding, consolidation, storage, and retrieval, representing the sequential steps through which information becomes part of one's memory.

Memory Priming: Enhanced ability to recall memory after exposure to related cues. Memory priming facilitates memory retrieval by exposure to stimuli or cues related to the target information.

Memory Recall: Retrieving information from memory storage. Memory recall involves returning stored information to conscious awareness, allowing individuals to remember and access previously learned material.

Memory Representation Phase: The initial step of committing information to memory by encoding it as mental representations. During the memory representation phase, information is transformed into mental images or concepts for storage in memory.

Memory Retrieval: Accessing information stored in memory. Memory retrieval is actively seeking and bringing forth stored information from memory storage.

Memory Retrieval Failure: Difficulty recalling information that is stored in memory. Memory retrieval failure occurs when information stored in memory is temporarily inaccessible or difficult to retrieve.

Memory Solution Phase: This stage of the memory process is where cues are used to search for target information. In the memory solution phase, individuals employ cues or prompts to aid in retrieving specific information from memory.

Memory Source Confusion: Recalling aspects of one memory while attributing them to another event or source of information. Memory source confusion involves the misattribution of details, leading to confusion about the origin of specific memories.

Memory Stimulation: Activating brain parts involved in memory using electrical or magnetic techniques. Memory stimulation techniques enhance memory function by directly influencing neural activity through electrical or magnetic stimulation.

Memory Suggestive Questioning: Cueing alters recollection of events, often unintentionally leading to false memories. Memory suggestive questioning involves prompts or questions that may inadvertently influence individuals' recollection of events, potentially leading to the formation of false memories.

Memory Support Systems: Tools and strategies for aiding or compensating for memory deficits. Memory support systems include various resources, such as organizational tools, reminders, and assistive technologies, designed to help individuals manage and cope with memory challenges.

Memory Technology Aids: Electronic devices that supplement memory, like smartwatches with reminders. Memory technology aids encompass a range of electronic devices and applications designed to assist individuals in managing and enhancing their memory function.

Method of Loci (Memory Palace): Memorization technique using visual-spatial cues based on familiar locations. The method of loci involves associating the information with specific areas in a familiar environment, facilitating memory recall by mentally retracing one's steps through these locations.

Mindfulness: Present-focused awareness and attention. It involves intentional, non-judgmental observation of the current moment, promoting mental well-being and cognitive benefits.

Misplaced Memories: Incorrectly recalling when or where a particular event occurred. Misplaced memories involve the distortion of temporal or spatial aspects of a memory, leading to inaccuracies in the recollection of when or where an event occurred.

Mnemonic Device: A memory aid like an acronym or rhyme to enhance encoding and recall. Mnemonic devices are memory-enhancing techniques that create associations or patterns to facilitate information retrieval. Acronyms and rhymes are common forms of mnemonic devices.

Mnemonics: Strategies for organizing information to make it more memorable. Mnemonics encompass various memory-enhancing techniques and strategies designed to aid in the encoding and retrieval of information by creating associations, patterns, or cues.

Mood Regulation: Controlling emotions through thoughts, behaviors, and activities. Mood regulation involves the conscious effort to manage and influence one's emotional well-being, which can impact cognitive processes, including memory.

Monoclonal Antibodies (mAbs): Laboratory-made proteins that target toxins like amyloid beta implicated in Alzheimer's. Monoclonal antibodies are synthetic proteins designed to specifically target and neutralize harmful substances, such as amyloid beta plaques, associated with Alzheimer's disease.

Multisensory Integration: Combining information from multiple senses to enhance memory encoding and retrieval. Multisensory integration involves the coordinated processing of information from different sensory modalities, contributing to more robust and effective memory formation.

N

Neural Circuits: Networks of interconnected neurons in the brain. Neural circuits represent interconnected pathways of neurons that work together to process and transmit information within the brain, contributing to various cognitive functions, including memory.

Neurofeedback: Using real-time displays of brain activity to teach self-regulation of cognition and emotions. Neurofeedback involves providing individuals with real-time information about their brain activity, allowing them to learn and regulate cognitive and emotional processes.

Neurogenesis: Generation of new neurons in specific brain regions like the hippocampus. Neurogenesis is the process by which new neurons are produced in specific regions of the brain, contributing to brain plasticity and potentially influencing memory and learning.

Neuroimaging: Visualizing and mapping brain structure and function using MRI, fMRI, PET, and CT scans. Neuroimaging techniques allow researchers to observe and analyze the structure and function of the brain, providing valuable insights into neural activity and memory processes.

Neurological Plasticity: Ability of the nervous system to rewire and adapt throughout life. Neurological plasticity, or neuroplasticity, refers to the brain's capacity to reorganize its structure and function in response to experience, learning, and environmental changes.

Neurological Rehabilitation: Therapies for relearning cognitive and motor skills after brain injury or disease. Neurological rehabilitation involves structured interventions and therapies aimed at helping individuals recover or adapt to cognitive and motor impairments resulting from brain injury or illness.

Neuroplasticity: Capacity of the brain to reorganize, form new connections, and change in response to experience. Neuroplasticity underscores the brain's ability to adapt, reorganize, and establish new relationships throughout life, influencing learning, memory, and cognitive functions.

Neuroscience: The interdisciplinary study of the brain and nervous system. Neuroscience encompasses the scientific exploration of the brain and nervous system, investigating their structure, function, and how they contribute to cognitive processes such as memory.

Neurotoxicity: Harmful effects of certain substances on nerve cells and signaling. Neurotoxicity refers to the damaging impact of substances on nerve cells, potentially affecting neural function, including memory processes.

Neurotransmitters: Chemicals like dopamine and acetylcholine that allow nerve cells to communicate. Neurotransmitters are chemical messengers that transmit signals between nerve cells, playing an essential role in synaptic communication and influencing cognitive functions, including memory.

Neuromodulation: Regulation of nerve activity through mechanisms that alter neurotransmitter release. Neuromodulation involves the adjustment of neural activity levels, often through the modulation of neurotransmitter release, impacting cognitive processes like memory.

Neuropsychologists: Psychologists who assess and treat cognitive, emotional, and behavioral disorders associated with the brain. Neuropsychologists specialize in evaluating and addressing disorders related to cognitive, emotional, and behavioral functioning, often stemming from brain-related conditions.

O

Oxidative Stress: Imbalance between free radicals and antioxidants that damage cells. Oxidative stress occurs when there is an imbalance between the production of free radicals, reactive oxygen species, and the body's ability to neutralize them with antioxidants, potentially impacting cellular health, including neurons.

P

Parietal Lobe: Part of the brain processes sensory information, attention, and spatial navigation. The parietal lobe plays a critical role in processing sensory information, spatial awareness, and directing attention, contributing to various cognitive functions, including memory.

Parkinson's Disease: Neurodegenerative disorder affecting movement as well as cognition and memory. Parkinson's disease is a progressive neurological disorder characterized by motor symptoms such as tremors and stiffness, but it can also impact cognitive functions, including memory.

PEMDAS: Mnemonic acronym for the order of operations in math: Parentheses, Exponents, Multiplication/Division, Addition/Subtraction. PEMDAS serves as a memory aid to help remember the order of mathematical operations: Parentheses, Exponents, Multiplication/Division, and Addition/Subtraction.

Pharmacological Interventions: Administering medications to improve symptoms or slow the progression of diseases like Alzheimer's. Pharmacological interventions involve the use of medications to manage symptoms or slow the progression of diseases, including those affecting memory, such as Alzheimer's.

Post-traumatic Stress Disorder (PTSD): A disorder involving intrusive memories, flashbacks, and avoidance behaviors after trauma. PTSD is a mental health condition that can result from exposure to traumatic events, often leading to symptoms such as intrusive memories and difficulties with memory processes.

Prospective Memory: Remembering to carry out future actions like taking medication or keeping appointments. Prospective memory involves remembering and executing planned actions in the future, such as fulfilling intentions or completing tasks at specific times.

Prospective Memory Aids: Tools like smart devices, alarms, and calendars that provide reminders and prompt intended actions. Prospective memory aids are external tools and cues designed to assist individuals in remembering and carrying out planned actions in the future.

Prospective Memory Failures: Lapses in remembering and completing intended tasks in the future. Prospective memory failures refer to instances where individuals experience difficulties remembering and successfully executing planned actions or tasks at specified future times.

Psychosocial Factors: Social, cultural, and psychological influences on cognition and memory over the lifespan. Psychosocial factors encompass the interplay of social, cultural, and psychological elements that can influence cognitive processes, including memory, throughout an individual's life.

Psychotropic Medications: Prescription drugs that affect brain chemicals and treat mental disorders, often with cognitive side effects. Psychotropic medications are drugs that impact brain chemistry and are prescribed to manage mental disorders, potentially influencing cognitive functions, including memory.

Pyramid Model of Memory: A model depicting sensory memory at the bottom, short-term memory in the middle, and long-term memory at the top. The pyramid model of memory conceptual

Psychedelics: Mind-altering substances like LSD and psilocybin that induce altered states of consciousness, perception, and cognition. They have a history of traditional use and are currently being researched for potential therapeutic applications in mental health conditions.

R

Recognition Memory Tests: Assessments of the ability to identify previously encountered items. These tests measure the capacity to recognize and acknowledge information or stimuli that have been previously learned or experienced.

Repression Therapy: A largely discontinued psychological treatment aimed at recovering repressed memories, often involving suggestion. This therapeutic approach, criticized for potential suggestion-induced false memories, sought to bring repressed memories to the conscious mind to address psychological issues.

Rivastigmine: An Alzheimer's medication that blocks the breakdown of acetylcholine to enhance cognitive function. It is used to manage symptoms of cognitive decline in conditions like Alzheimer's disease.

Roy G. Biv: A mnemonic for remembering the sequence of hues in the color spectrum - Red, Orange, Yellow, Green, Blue, Indigo, Violet.

S

Selective Memory: The tendency to have a better memory for experiences that confirm biases and existing beliefs. It involves remembering information that aligns with pre-existing attitudes or beliefs while selectively forgetting or downplaying contradictory information.

Sense of Identity: One's conception and expression of individuality and selfhood constructed from experiences and memory. It encompasses the subjective awareness of being a unique and continuous entity over time.

Sensory & Physical Skills Tests: Neuropsychological assessments evaluating perceptual abilities and motor function. These tests measure the integrity of sensory and motor pathways, providing insights into an individual's physical and sensory capabilities.

Sensory Memory: Very brief storage of sensory information from sight, hearing, smell, taste, and touch. It represents the initial stage of memory, where sensory input is briefly retained before being transferred to short-term memory.

Semantic Memory Tests: Assessments of general factual knowledge like vocabulary, concepts, and trivia. These tests evaluate the recall of general knowledge and information about the world.

Serotonin and Endorphins: Neurotransmitters regulating mood, well-being, learning, memory, and motivation. Serotonin contributes to mood regulation, and endorphins act as natural painkillers and mood enhancers.

Short-Term Memory Tests: Evaluations of temporary memory storage capacity, typically for spans of 5-9 items. These tests assess an individual's ability to hold and manipulate information temporarily.

Sleep Disturbances: Disruptions in sleep quality and patterns that can impair memory consolidation. Sleep disturbances, including insomnia or sleep disorders, may adversely affect the forming and storing of memories.

Sleep Environment: Physical surroundings, noise, light, temperature, and other factors impacting sleep quality. The sleep environment is fundamental in promoting restful sleep, which is essential for memory consolidation.

Source Amnesia: Forgetting the source of remembered information or memories. It involves the inability to recall where or how a particular information was acquired.

Source Confusion: Difficulty distinguishing how, when, or where memory was acquired due to similarities between sources. This can lead to errors in attributing memories to the wrong source.

Spinal Fluid Tests: Analyzing cerebrospinal fluid via lumbar puncture to detect dementia-related biomarkers. These tests provide valuable diagnostic information about conditions affecting the central nervous system, including dementia.

Stem Cell Therapy: Introducing stem cells to repair damage and induce regeneration in the brain to treat cognitive decline. This emerging therapeutic approach aims to harness the regenerative potential of stem cells to address neurological disorders.

Stress and Cognitive Load: Impact of strain on the brain's capacity to process information and form memories. Anxiety and cognitive load can negatively affect cognitive functions, including memory.

Stress Management: Techniques and practices for regulating the mind-body stress response and mitigating harmful effects on cognition. Stress management strategies aim to reduce the impact of stressors on mental and physical well-being.

Stress Resilience: Capacity to cope and adapt to stressors in ways that preserve functioning and well-being. Stress resilience involves maintaining psychological and physiological balance in challenging situations.

Structural Brain Changes: Alterations in gray matter, white matter, and ventricles associated with memory disorders and dementia. These changes in brain structure are often observed in conditions that impact memory function, such as Alzheimer's disease.

T

Temporal Lobe: A brain region that processes sensory input, comprehends language, forms memories, and regulates emotion. It is essential in various cognitive functions, including memory formation and language comprehension.

Thyroid Hormones: Thyroxine and triiodothyronine hormones regulate metabolism and impact neural function. These hormones play a role in maintaining overall physiological health, and disruptions in thyroid function can affect cognitive processes, including memory.

Tip-of-the-Tongue (TOT) Phenomenon: Temporary inability to recall information that feels on the verge of being remembered. It is a common experience where an individual knows the information is stored in memory but struggles to retrieve it.

Traumatic Brain Injuries (TBIs): Head injuries causing cognitive dysfunction like attentional deficits and memory impairment. TBIs can have varying effects on memory, depending on the severity and location of the injury in the brain.

Transcranial Direct Current Stimulation (tDCS): A form of neuromodulation applying a weak constant electric current to the brain via electrodes. It modulates neural activity and has been explored as a potential cognitive enhancement and memory improvement intervention.

Transcranial Magnetic Stimulation (TMS): Noninvasive brain stimulation using rapidly changing magnetic fields to induce electrical currents. TMS is a technique used to modulate neural activity and has applications in studying brain function and treating certain neurological conditions.

V

Vascular Dementia: Dementia results from reduced brain blood flow due to stroke or artery blockages. It is a type of dementia caused by problems with the blood supply to the brain, leading to cognitive decline.

Vascular Factors: Conditions affecting blood vessels and circulation that influence dementia risk. Health factors such as hypertension and atherosclerosis can contribute to vascular dementia.

Virtual Reality (VR) and Augmented Reality (AR): Computer-generated simulations of real-world environments and overlaying digital information onto natural settings. These technologies have been used in memory research and rehabilitation, creating immersive experiences for cognitive training.

Visual Memory: Memory related to recognizing, recalling, and manipulating visual information and imagery. Visual memory is essential for recognizing faces, remembering locations, and recalling graphic details.

W

Wernicke-Korsakoff Syndrome: Disorder causing memory loss often associated with alcohol misuse and thiamine deficiency. It is a neurological disorder resulting from a thiamine deficiency (vitamin B1) characterized by severe memory impairment.

Working Memory: System for temporarily storing and manipulating information for cognitive tasks. Working memory is crucial for tasks that require the temporary retention and manipulation of information, such as problem-solving and comprehension.

References

Alzheimer's Association. (2021). FDA-Approved Treatments for Alzheimer's.

Alzheimer's & Dementia: (2020). Translational Research & Clinical Interventions, 10.1002/trc2.12028, 6, 1.

Alzheimer's Society. (2019, May 17). Changes in Behavior.

Akhter, F., Persaud, A., Zaokari, Y., Zhao, Z., & Zhu, D. (2021). Vascular dementia and underlying sex differences. Frontiers in Aging Neuroscience, 13, 720715.

Ali SA, Begum T, Reza F. Hormonal Influences on Cognitive Function. Malays J Med Sci. 2018 Jul;25(4):31-41. doi: 10.21315/mjms2018.25.4.3. Epub 2018 Aug 30. PMID: 30914845; PMCID: PMC6422548.

Ali, S. M., & Singh, S. B. (2023). A brief review on the potential of psychedelics for treating Alzheimer's disease and related depression. Frontiers in Psychiatry, 14, 1059943. doi:10.3389/fpsyt.2023.1059943

Andrade, A. G., Bubu, O. M., Varga, A. W., & Osorio, R. S. (2018). The Relationship between Obstructive Sleep Apnea and Alzheimer's Disease. Journal of Alzheimer's Disease: JAD, 64(s1), S255–S270.

American Heart Association. (2018). How Much Physical Activity Do You Need?

Beam, C. R., Kaneshiro, C., Jang, J. Y., Reynolds, C. A., Pedersen, N. L., & Gatz, M. (2018). Differences Between Women and Men in Incidence Rates of Dementia and Alzheimer's Disease. Journal of Alzheimer's Disease,64(4), 1077-1083.

Beckley Foundation, The (2023). LSD and creativity: Increased novelty, symbolic thinking, decreased utility, and convergent thinking.

Bediou, B., Adams, D. M., Mayer, R. E., Tipton, E., Green, C. S., & Bavelier, D. (2018). Meta-analysis of action video game impact on perceptual, attentional, and cognitive skills. Psychological Bulletin, 144(1), 77-110.

Belleville, S., Clement, F., Mellah, S., Gilbert, B., Fontaine, F., & Gauthier, S. (2018). Training-related brain plasticity in subjects at risk of developing Alzheimer's disease. Brain, 141(3), 841-857.

Belleville, S., Chertkow, H., Gauthier, S., & De Rosa, M. (2007). The neuropsychology of Alzheimer's disease. In D. T. Stuss & R. T. Knight (Eds.), Principles of Frontal Lobe Function (pp. 565-586). Oxford University Press.

Benvenuti, M., Giovagnoli, S., Mazzoni, E., Cipresso, P., Pedroli, E., & Riva, G. (2020). The Relevance of Online Social Relationships Among the Elderly: How Using the Web Could Enhance Quality of Life? Frontiers in Psychology, 11, 551862.

Bisht, K., Sharma, K., & Tremblay, M. (2018). Chronic stress as a risk factor for Alzheimer's disease: Roles of microglia-mediated synaptic remodeling, inflammation, and oxidative stress. Neurobiology of Stress,9, 9-21.

Bisht, K., Sharma, K., & Tremblay, M. (2018). Chronic stress as a risk factor for Alzheimer's disease: Roles of microglia-mediated synaptic remodeling, inflammation, and oxidative stress. Neurobiology of Stress, 9, 9-21.

Biderman, N., & Shohamy, D. (2021). Memory and decision-making interact to shape the value of unchosen options. Nat Commun, 12, 4648.

Bir, S. C., Khan, M. W., Javalkar, V., Toledo, E. G., & Kelley, R. E. (2021). Emerging concepts in vascular dementia: A review. Journal of Stroke and Cerebrovascular Diseases, 30(8), 105864.

Bischof, G. N., & Park, D. C. (2015). Obesity and Aging: Consequences for Cognition, Brain Structure and Brain Function. Psychosomatic medicine, 77(6), 697.

Bloom, G. S. (2014). Amyloid-β and Tau: The Trigger and Bullet in Alzheimer Disease Pathogenesis. JAMA Neurology, 71(4), 505.

Bopp, K. L., & Verhaeghen, P. (2021). Working memory and aging: A meta-analysis. Journal of Gerontology: Psychological Sciences, 76(2), 281-293.

Boada, M., Lopez, O., Nunez, L., Szczepiorkowski, Z. M., Torres, M., Grifols, C., Paez, A., & The Alzheimer's Disease and Thrombosis Forum. (2019). Plasma exchange for Alzheimer's disease Management by Albumin Replacement (AMBAR) trial: Study design and progress. Alzheimer's & Dementia: Translational Research & Clinical Interventions, 5, 61–69.

Brennan, Dan. (2021, March 18). Learning after 60. WebMD.

BrightFocus Foundation. (2021, August 25). Healthy aging: Cognitive reserve and how to Strengthen it.

Bruggeman, G. F., Haitsma, I. K., F. Dirven, C. M., & Volovici, V. (2020). Traumatic axonal injury (TAI): Definitions, pathophysiology, and imaging—A narrative review. Acta Neurochirurgica, 163(1), 31-44.

Burtscher, J., Mallet, R. T., Burtscher, M., & Millet, G. P. (2021). Hypoxia and brain aging: Neurodegeneration or neuroprotection? Ageing Research Reviews, 68, 101343.

Carhart-Harris, R., & Friston, K. J. (2023). The potential of psychedelics for treating mental health disorders. Biological Psychiatry, 94(10), 904-914. doi: 10.1016/j.biopsych.2022.08.008

CDC, S. (2022, May 21). The effects of diabetes on the brain. Centers for Disease Control and Prevention.

Centers for Disease Control and Prevention. (2020). Memory and Cognitive Impairment.

Cleeland, C., Pipingas, A., Scholey, A., & White, D. (2019). Neurochemical changes in the aging brain: A systematic review. Neuroscience & Biobehavioral Reviews, 98, 306–319.

Cowansage, K. K. et al. Direct reactivation of a coherent neocortical memory of context. Neuron, 84, 432–441.

Crary, J. F., Trojanowski, J. Q., Schneider, J. A., Abisambra, J. F., Abner, E. L., Alafuzoff, I., ... & Bennett, D. A. (2014). Primary age-related tauopathy (PART): a common pathology associated with human aging. Acta Neuropathologica, 128(6), 755-766.

Davis, L., & Miller, S. (2023). The Role of Gene Therapy in Brain Care. Genetics and Medicine, 14(2), 89-100.

de Souza-Talarico JN, Marin MF, Sindi S, Lupien SJ. Effects of stress hormones on the brain and cognition: Evidence from normal to pathological aging. Dement Neuropsychol. 2011 Jan-Mar;5(1):8-16. doi: 10.1590/S1980-57642011DN05010003. PMID: 29213714; PMCID: PMC5619133.

Delli Pizzi S, Chiacchiaretta P, Sestieri C, Ferretti A, Tullo MG, Della Penna S, Martinotti G, Onofrj M, Roseman L, Timmermann C, Nutt DJ, Carhart-Harris RL, Sensi SLet al., 2023, LSD-induced changes in the functional connectivity of distinct thalamic nuclei., Neuroimage, Vol: 283

DeNardo, L. A. et al. Temporal evolution of cortical ensembles promoting remote memory retrieval. Nat. Neurosci., 22, 460–469.

Dings, R., & Newen, A. (2023). Constructing the past: The relevance of the narrative self in modulating episodic memory. Rev.Phil. Psych, 25, 36-46.

Dixon, R. A., & de Frias, C. M. (2014). The Victoria Longitudinal Study: From characterizing cognitive aging to illustrating changes in memory compensation. Aging, Neuropsychology, and Cognition, 21(3), 331-365.

Doan, S. N., Finogenov, I., Elbaz, M., & Gaysina, D. (2019). Associations between psychological well-being and cognitive performance in older adults. Journal of Aging Research, 5(7), 1-14.

Dragan, A. L. (2022). Memory and Stress in Later Life: A Review. Journal of the American Geriatrics Society, 70(1), 35-43.

Dunlavey CJ. Introduction to the Hypothalamic-Pituitary-Adrenal Axis: Healthy and Dysregulated Stress Responses, Developmental Stress and Neurodegeneration. J Undergrad Neurosci Educ. 2018 Jun 15;16(2): R59-R60. PMID: 30057514; PMCID: PMC6057754.

Elder, C. L. (2020). The Brain and How it Ages. Nova Science Publishers, Inc.

Fiorenzato, E., Strafella, A. P., Kim, J., Schifano, R., Weis, L., Antonini, A., & Biundo, R. (2021). Dynamic functional connectivity changes associated with dementia in Parkinson's disease. Brain, 144(8), 2309-2320.

FDA. (2021). FDA's Decision to Approve New Treatment for Alzheimer's Disease.

Fogel, S. M., Albouy, G., King, B. R., Lungu, O., Vien, C., Bore, A., ... & Doyon, J. (2019). Reactivation or transformation? Motor cortical plasticity for motor sequence learning. Journal of Neuroscience, 39(29), 5675-5686.

Foo, F. (2019). Current treatments for cognitive decline in the elderly. The Lancet Neurology, 18(4), 339-340.

Fritz, J., Mishkin, M. & Saunders, R. C. In search of an auditory engram. Proc. Natl Acad. Sci. USA, 102, 9359–9364.

Gajewski, P. D., & Falkenstein, M. (2016). Physical activity and neurocognitive functioning in aging a condensed updated review. European Review of Aging and Physical Activity, 13(1), 1-7.

Garcia-Romeu, A., & Rosenberg, P. B. (2023, April 19). Can psychedelics help patients with dementia? Penn Memory Center.

Gates, N., Fiatarone Singh, M. A., Sachdev, P. S., & Valenzuela, M. (2013). The effect of exercise training on cognitive function in older adults with mild cognitive impairment: a meta-analysis of randomized controlled trials. The American Journal of Geriatric Psychiatry, 21(11), 1086–1097.

Gauthier, S., Leuzy, A., Racine, E., & Rosa-Neto, P. (2013). Diagnosis and management of Alzheimer's disease: Past, present, and future ethical issues. Progress in Neurobiology, 110, 102-113.

Gerstorf, D., Lövdén, M., Röcke, C., Smith, J., & Lindenberger, U. (2007). Well-being affects changes in perceptual speed in advanced old age: Longitudinal evidence for a dynamic link. Developmental psychology, 43(3), 705.

Gobel, E. W., Parrish, T. B., & Reber, P. J. (2011). Neural correlates of skill acquisition: Decreased cortical activity during a serial interception sequence learning task. Neuroimage, 58(4), 1150-1157.

Green, C. S., & Bavelier, D. (2008). Exercising your brain: A review of human brain plasticity and training-induced learning. Psychology and Aging, 23(4), 692.

Gustafsson, A., Strömberg, H., Kallin, K., & Nyberg, L. (2019). Neurocognitive Effects of Cognitive Training in Older Adults. The Gerontologist, 59(2), 282-292.

Haeger, A., Costa, A. S., Schulz, J. B., & Reetz, K. (2020). Exploring the multidimensional complex systems structure of the stress response and its relation to health and sleep outcomes. Brain, Behavior, and Immunity, 89, 867-879.

Han, J. H. et al. Selective erasure of a fear memory. Science, 323, 1492–1496.

Helmstetter, F. J., Parsons, R. G. & Gafford, G. M. Macromolecular synthesis, distributed synaptic plasticity, and fear conditioning. Neurobiol. Learn. Mem., 89, 324–337.

Hertzog, C., Kramer, A. F., Wilson, R. S., & Lindenberger, U. (2008). Enrichment Effects on Adult Cognitive Development: Can the Functional Capacity of Older Adults Be Preserved and Enhanced? Psychological Science in the Public Interest, 9(1), 1-65.

Hebb, D. O. The Organization of Behavior; A Neuropsychological Theory (Wiley, 1949).

Hosseini, S., Maillard, P., & Madison, C. M. (2022). State-of-the-art imaging techniques for the diagnosis of early-stage Alzheimer's. Journal of Neurology, Neurosurgery & Psychiatry, 93(1), 101-110.

Hunter, L. E., & Bachman, D. L. (2019). Cognitive impairment and dementia in Parkinson's disease. Handbook of Clinical Neurology, 167, 349-364.

Iwasa, H., Gondo, Y., Yoshida, Y., Kwon, J., Inagaki, H., & Kawaai, C. (2008). Cognitive Performance as a Predictor of Functional Decline Among the Non-disabled Elderly Dwelling in a Japanese Community: A 4-Year Population-Based Prospective Cohort Study. Archives of Gerontology and Geriatrics, 47(1), 139-149.

Jagger, C., Matthews, R., Melzer, D., Matthews, F., Brayne, C., & MRC CFAS. (2007). Educational differences in the dynamics of disability incidence, recovery, and mortality: Findings from the MRC Cognitive Function and Ageing Study (MRC CFAS). International journal of epidemiology, 36(2), 358-365.

Johns Hopkins Center for Psychedelic and Consciousness Research. Johns Hopkins Medicine, (2023)

Johnson, N. F., Kim, C., & Clasey, J. L. (2012). The influence of exercise on cognitive abilities. Comprehensive Physiology, 2(1), 403-428.

Josselyn, S. A., Kohler, S. & Frankland, P. W. Finding the engram. Nat. Rev. Neurosci., 16, 521–534.

Jurado, M. B., & Rosselli, M. (2007). The elusive nature of executive functions: A review of our current understanding. Neuropsychology Review, 17(3), 213-233.

Justice, N. J. (2018). The relationship between stress and Alzheimer's disease. Neurobiology of Stress, 8, 127-133.

Karr, J. E., Areshenkoff, C. N., & Garcia-Barrera, M. A. (2014). The neuropsychological outcomes of concussion: A systematic review of meta-analyses on the cognitive sequelae of mild traumatic brain injury. Neuropsychology, 28(3), 321.

Kerkar, S. P., Das, A., & Vaz, A. (2019). Cognitive decline and quality of life in the elderly. Journal of Gerontology, 6(2), 33-37.

Kerr, D. S., Cheng, S. Y., Gomes, F. V., & Grace, A. A. (2022). Long-term consequences of stress on age-related cognitive decline. Neurobiology of Stress, 15, 100412.

Khadilkar SV, Patil VA. Sex Hormones and Cognition: Where Do We Stand? J Obstet Gynaecol India. 2019 Aug;69(4):303-312. doi: 10.1007/s13224-019-01223-5. Epub 2019 Apr 10. PMID: 31391735; PMCID: PMC6661054.

Kirson, N. Y., Meadows, E. S., Desai, U., Smith, B. P., Cheung, H. C., Zuckerman, P., Matthews, B. R. (2019). Temporal and Geographic Variation in the Incidence of Alzheimer's Disease Diagnosis in the US between 2007 and 2014. Journal of the American Geriatrics Society, 68(2), 346-353.

Kitamura, T. et al. Engrams and circuits crucial for systems consolidation of a memory. Science, 356, 73–78.

Kuh, D., Cooper, R., Hardy, R., Richards, M., & Ben-Shlomo, Y. (2014). A life course approach to healthy aging. Oxford University Press.

Lech, R. K., & Suchan, B. (2013). The medial temporal lobe: Memory and beyond. Behavioral brain research, 254, 45-49.

Li, R., Singh, M., & Singh, S. (2019). Cerebrovascular diseases and cognitive impairment. Neurodegenerative Disease Management, 9(2), 63-77.

Li, S. C., Schmiedek, F., Huxhold, O., Röcke, C., Smith, J., & Lindenberger, U. (2008). Working memory plasticity in old age: practice gain, transfer, and maintenance. Psychology and Aging, 23(4), 731.

Lieberman, J. A., Dunbar, G., Segreti, A. C., Girgis, R. R., Seoane, F., Beaver, J. S., ... & Hosford, D. A. (2013). A randomized exploratory trial of an alpha-7 nicotinic receptor agonist (TC-5619) for cognitive enhancement in schizophrenia. Neuropsychopharmacology, 38(6), 968-975.

Liu, X. et al. Optogenetic stimulation of a hippocampal engram activates fear memory recall. Nature, 484, 381–385.

Loprinzi, P. D., & Frith, E. (2018). A brief primer on the mediational role of BDNF in the exercise-memory link. Clinical physiology and functional imaging, 38(1), 9-14.

Lustig, C., Shah, P., Seidler, R., & Reuter-Lorenz, P. A. (2009). Aging, training, and the brain: A review and future directions. Neuropsychology review, 19(4), 504-522.

Mackenzie, I. R. (2018). The neuropathology and clinical phenotype of FTD with progranulin mutations. Acta neuropathologica, 116(1), 63-77.

Mayo Clinic. (2019, April 19). Dementia.

Maguire, E. A., Gadian, D. G., Johnsrude, I. S., Good, C. D., Ashburner, J., Frackowiak, R. S., & Frith, C. D. (2000). Navigation-related structural change in the hippocampi of taxi drivers. Proceedings of the National Academy of Sciences, 97(8), 4398-4403.

Matthews, K. A., Xu, W., Gaglioti, A. H., Holt, J. B., Croft, J. B., Mack, D., & Mcguire, L. C. (2018). Racial and ethnic estimates of Alzheimer's disease and related dementias in the United States (2015-2060) in adults aged ≥65 years. Alzheimer's & Dementia, 21(1), 17-24.

Manning, K. J., Clarke, C., Lorry, A., Weintraub, D., Wilkinson, J. R., Duda, J. E., ... & Stern, M. B. (2016). Medication management and neuropsychological performance in Parkinson's disease. The Clinical Neuropsychologist, 30(7), 1087-1100.

Maruff P, Falleti M. Cognitive function in growth hormone deficiency and growth hormone replacement. Horm Res. 2005;64 Suppl 3:100-8. doi: 10.1159/000089325. Epub 2006 Jan 20. PMID: 16439852.

Mayo Clinic. (2021). Memory Loss: When to Seek Help.

McGaugh, J. L., & Roozendaal, B. (2002). Role of adrenal stress hormones in forming lasting memories in the brain. Current opinion in neurobiology, 12(2), 205-210.

Mirelman, A., Bonato, P., & Camicioli, R. (2019). Gait impairments in Parkinson's disease. The Lancet Neurology, 18(7), 697-708.

THE TAPESTRY OF MEMORY: UNRAVELING THE THREADS OF THE MIND

Miura, H., Ozaki, N., Sawada, M., Isobe, K., Ohta, T., & Nagatsu, T. (2008). A link between stress and depression: Shifts in the balance between the kynurenine and serotonin pathways of tryptophan metabolism and the etiology and pathophysiology of depression. Stress, 11(3), 198-209.

Mizumori, S. J. Y., & Jo, Y. S. (2013). Homeostatic regulation of memory systems and adaptive decisions. Hippocampus, 23(11), 1103-1124.

Moreno-Jiménez, E. P., Flor-García, M., Terreros-Roncal, J., Rábano, A., Cafini, F., Pallas-Bazarra, N., ... & Llorens-Martín, M. (2019). Adult hippocampal neurogenesis is abundant in neurologically healthy subjects and drops sharply in patients with Alzheimer's disease. Nature Medicine, 25(4), 554-560.

Morris, M. C., Tangney, C. C., Wang, Y., Sacks, F. M., Bennett, D. A., & Aggarwal, N. T. (2015). MIND diet associated with reduced incidence of Alzheimer's disease. Alzheimer's & dementia: The Journal of the Alzheimer's Association, 11(9), 1007–1014.

Mostert, J. C., & Koch, S. B. (2017). The role of early life stress in HPA axis and anxiety. Advances in experimental medicine and biology, 1010, 147-160.

Müller, F., Mithoefer, M. C., & Liechti, M. E. (2023). Pharmacological and clinical aspects of psychedelics: A review of human studies. Pharmacological Reviews, 75(3), 414-445. doi:10.1124/pharmrev.121.000846

Nadel, L., & Moscovitch, M. (1997). Memory consolidation, retrograde amnesia, and the hippocampal complex. Current opinion in neurobiology, 7(2), 217-227.

National Institute on Aging. (2021). Memory, Forgetfulness, and Aging: What's Normal and What's Not?

National Institute of Aging. (2019, June 13). Alzheimer's Disease Fact Sheet

National Institute of Aging. (2015, May 14). What are the Signs of Alzheimer's Disease?

Neuroscience News (March 31, 2023) The cognitive benefits of psychedelics.

Niemann, C., Godde, B., & Voelcker-Rehage, C. (2014). Cardiovascular and coordinative exercise increases hippocampal volume in older adults—frontiers in aging neuroscience, 6, 170.

National Institute of Neurological Disorders and Stroke. (2019, June 16), The Dementias: Hope Through Research.

Nithianantharajah, J., & Hannan, A. J. (2009). Enriched environments, experience-dependent plasticity, and disorders of the nervous system. Nature Reviews Neuroscience, 7(9), 697-709.

Nutt DJ, 2023, Pharmacological Dissection of Antipsychotics, BIOLOGICAL PSYCHIATRY, Vol: 94, Pages: 524-525, ISSN: 0006-3223

Ohkawa, N. et al. Artificial association of pre-stored information to generate a qualitatively new memory. Cell Rep., 11, 261–269.

Öhman, H., Savikko, N., Strandberg, T. E., & Pitkälä, K. H. (2014). Effect of Physical Exercise on Cognitive Performance in Older Adults with Mild Cognitive Impairment or Dementia: A Systematic Review. Dementia and Geriatric Cognitive Disorders, 38(5-6), 347-365.

Olsson, A., Csajbok, L., Ost, M., Höglund, K., Nylén, K., Rosengren, L., ... & Blenn

Ow, K. (2004). Marked increase of β-amyloid1-42 and amyloid precursor protein in ventricular cerebrospinal fluid after severe traumatic brain injury. Journal of Neurology, 251(7), 870-876.

Owen, A. M., Morris, R. G., Sahakian, B. J., Polkey, C. E., & Robbins, T. W. (1996). Double dissociation of memory and executive functions in working memory tasks following frontal lobe excisions, temporal lobe excisions, or amygdalo-hippocampectomy in man. Brain, 119(5), 1597-1616.

Palmqvist, S., Schöll, M., Strandberg, O., Mattsson, N., Stomrud, E., Zetterberg, H., ... & Hansson, O. (2019). Earliest accumulation of β-amyloid occurs within the default-mode network and concurrently affects brain connectivity. Nature Communications, 10(1), 1-12.

Panenka, W. J., Lange, R. T., Bouix, S., Shewchuk, J. R., Heran, M. K., Brubacher, J. R., ... & Iverson, G. L. (2015). Neuropsychological outcome and diffusion tensor imaging in complicated versus uncomplicated mild traumatic brain injury. PloS one, 10(4), e0122746.

Papez, J. W. (1937). A proposed mechanism of emotion. Archives of Neurology & Psychiatry, 38(4), 725-743.

Park, J. H., Lee, S. B., Lee, T. J., Lee, D. Y., Jhoo, J. H., Youn, J. C., ... & Woo, J. I. (2011). Depression in vascular dementia is quantitatively and qualitatively different from depression in Alzheimer's disease. Dementia and geriatric cognitive disorders, 31(4), 272-277.

Pereira, A. C., Huddleston, D. E., Brickman, A. M., Sosunov, A. A., Hen, R., McKhann, G. M., ... & Small, S. A. (2007). An in vivo correlate of exercise-induced neurogenesis in the adult dentate gyrus. Proceedings of the National Academy of Sciences, 104(13), 5638-5643.

Petersen, R. C., Smith, G. E., Waring, S. C., Ivnik, R. J., Tangalos, E. G., & Kokmen, E. (1999). Mild cognitive impairment: clinical characterization and outcome. Archives of Neurology, 56(3), 303-308.

Petzold, A., Psotta, L., Brigadski, T., Endres, T., & Lessmann, V. (2015). Chronic BDNF deficiency leads to an age-dependent impairment in spatial learning. Neurobiology of learning and memory, 120, 52-60.

Plassman, B. L., Langa, K. M., Fisher, G. G., Heeringa, S. G., Weir, D. R., Ofstedal, M. B., ... & Wallace, R. B. (2007). Prevalence of dementia in the United States: the aging, demographics, and memory study. Neuroepidemiology, 29(1-2), 125-132.

Possin, K. L., Chester, S. K., LaMarre, A. K., & Geschwind, M. D. (2013). The frontal-anatomy-based naming test. Journal of the International Neuropsychological Society, 19(3), 335.

Priede. Ph.D., David; Ylagan, Camille; Fernando, Thinuri; Khan, Salma; Krishnan, Saksha; Artamendi, Sophia. The Conditions Afflicting the Body, Mind, and Soul of America (p. 454). BioLife Publishing. Kindle Edition.

Qin, Y. L., McNaughton, B. L., Skaggs, W. E., & Barnes, C. A. (1997). Memory reprocessing in corticocortical and hippocampocortical neuronal ensembles. Philosophical Transactions of the Royal Society of London. Series B: Biological Sciences, 352(1360), 1525-1533.

Rampon, C., Tang, Y. P., Goodhouse, J., Shimizu, E., Kyin, M., & Tsien, J. Z. (2000). Enrichment induces structural changes and recovery from nonspatial memory deficits in CA1 NMDAR1-knockout mice. Nature Neuroscience, 3(3), 238-244.

Rapp, P. R., & Amaral, D. G. (1989). Evidence for task-dependent memory dysfunction in the aged monkey. Journal of Neuroscience, 9(10), 3568-3576.

Rapp, P. R., & Gallagher, M. (1996). Preserved neuron number in the hippocampus of aged rats with spatial learning deficits. Proceedings of the National Academy of Sciences, 93(18), 9926-9930.

Rascovsky, K. (2016, July/August). A Primer in Neuropsychological Assessment for Dementia. July 6, 2020,

Rauschecker, J. P., & Scott, S. K. (2009). Maps and streams in the auditory cortex: nonhuman primates illuminate human speech processing. Nature Neuroscience, 12(6), 718-724.

Redondo, R. L. et al. Bidirectional switch of the valence associated with a hippocampal contextual memory engram. Nature, 513, 426–430.

Robert, P., & Onyike, C. U. (2013). Frontotemporal dementia. The Lancet, 382(9904), 1662-1671.

Rosen, A. C., Gabrieli, J. D., Stoub, T., Prull, M. W., O'Hara, R., Friedman, L., ... & deToledo-Morrell, L. (2005). Relating medial temporal lobe volume to frontal fMRI activation for memory encoding in older adults. Cortex, 41(4), 595-602.

Rosenblum, W. I. (2014). Why Alzheimer trials fail: removing soluble oligomeric beta-amyloid is essential, inconsistent, and difficult. Neurobiology of aging, 35(5), 969-974.

Rosenzweig, E. S., & Barnes, C. A. (2003). Impact of aging on hippocampal function: plasticity, network dynamics, and cognition. Progress in neurobiology, 69(3), 143-179.

Rossor, M. N., Fox, N. C., Mummery, C. J., Schott, J. M., & Warren, J. D. (2010). The diagnosis of young-onset dementia. The Lancet Neurology, 9(8), 793-806.

Roy, D. S. et al. Distinct neural circuits for the formation and retrieval of episodic memories. Cell, 170, 1000–1012.

Rovee-Collier, C., & Cuevas, K. (2009). Multiple memory systems are unnecessary to account for infant memory development: an ecological model. Developmental psychology, 45(1), 160.

Ruben, J., Schwiemann, J., Deuchert, M., Meyer, R., Krause, T., Curio, G., ... & Villringer, A. (2001). Somatotopic organization of the human secondary somatosensory cortex. Cerebral Cortex, 11(5), 463-473.

Rugg, M. D., & Vilberg, K. L. (2013). Brain networks underlying episodic memory retrieval. Current opinion in neurobiology, 23(2), 255-260.

Rygiel, K. (2016). Novel strategies for Alzheimer's disease treatment: An overview of anti-amyloid beta monoclonal antibodies. Indian Journal of Pharmacology,48(6), 629.

Rygiel, K. (2016). Novel strategies for Alzheimer's disease treatment: An overview of anti-amyloid beta monoclonal antibodies. Indian Journal of Pharmacology, 48(6), 629.

Rypma, B., & D'Esposito, M. (2000). Isolating the neural mechanisms of age-related changes in human working memory. Nature Neuroscience, 3(5), 509-515.

Sacks, O. (1985). The man who mistook his wife for a hat and other clinical tales. Simon and Schuster.

Saeger, J. B., & Olson, D. E. (2023). The potential of psychedelics for the treatment of Alzheimer's disease and related dementias. Pharmacological Reviews, 75(3), 564-588. doi:10.1124/pharmrev.121.000856

Sahay, A., Scobie, K. N., Hill, A. S., O'Carroll, C. M., Kheirbek, M. A., Burghardt, N. S., ... & Hen, R. (2011). Increasing adult hippocampal neurogenesis is sufficient to improve pattern separation. Nature, 472(7344), 466-470.

Salthouse, T. A. (2009). When does age-related cognitive decline begin? Neurobiology of aging, 30(4), 507-514.

Saper, C. B., Scammell, T. E., & Lu, J. (2005). Hypothalamic regulation of sleep and circadian rhythms. Nature, 437(7063), 1257-1263.

Satoh, M., Takeda, K., Nagata, I., Kuzuhara, S., & Yokota, T. (2011). A comparative study of radiological findings between dementia with Lewy bodies and Alzheimer's disease. Brain Research, 1369, 13-22.

Saykin, A. J., Wishart, H. A., Rabin, L. A., Santulli, R. B., Flashman, L. A., West, J. D., ... & Mamourian, A. C. (2006). Older adults with cognitive complaints show brain atrophy similar to that of amnestic MCI. Neurology, 67(5), 834-842.

Schaefer, S. Y., & Duff, K. (2015). Rapid responsiveness to practice predicts longer-term retention of upper extremity motor skills in non-demented older adults. Frontiers in aging neuroscience, 7, 214.

Schaie, K. W. (1994). The course of adult intellectual development. American psychologist, 49(4), 304.

Scheltens, P., Fox, N., Barkhof, F., & De Carli, C. (2002). Structural magnetic resonance imaging in the practical assessment of dementia: beyond exclusion. The Lancet Neurology, 1(1), 13-21.

Schmitter-Edgecombe, M., Woo, E., & Greeley, D. R. (2009). Characterizing multiple memory deficits and their relation to everyday functioning in individuals with mild cognitive impairment. Neuropsychology, 23(2), 168.

Schulz, R., & Martire, L. M. (2004). Family caregiving of persons with dementia: prevalence, health effects, and support strategies. The American journal of geriatric psychiatry, 12(3), 240-249.

Schwartz, M. W., Woods, S. C., Porte, D., Seeley, R. J., & Baskin, D. G. (2000). Central nervous system control of food intake. Nature, 404(6778), 661-671.

Scoville, W. B., & Milner, B. (1957). Loss of recent memory after bilateral hippocampal lesions. Journal of Neurology, Neurosurgery & Psychiatry, 20(1), 11-21.

Sheline, Y. I., Raichle, M. E., Snyder, A. Z., Morris, J. C., Head, D., Wang, S., & Mintun, M. A. (2010). Amyloid plaques disrupt resting state default mode network connectivity in cognitively normal elderly. Biological psychiatry, 67(6), 584-587.

Shepherd, J. D., & Bear, M. F. (2011). New views of Arc, a master regulator of synaptic plasticity. Nature Neuroscience, 14(3), 279-284.

Sherwin, B. B. (2003). Estrogen and cognitive functioning in women. Endocrine Reviews, 24(2), 133-151.

Siddique, H., & Yount, G. (2012). The role of dietary supplements in cognitive enhancement. Nutrition and dietary supplements, 4, 85-95.

Singh, S. K., Srivastav, S., Castellani, R. J., Plascencia-Villa, G., & Perry, G. (2019). Neuroprotective and Antioxidant Effect of Ginkgo biloba Extract Against AD and Other Neurological Disorders. Neurotherapeutics, 16(3), 666-674.

Small, S. A., Schobel, S. A., Buxton, R. B., Witter, M. P., & Barnes, C. A. (2011). A pathophysiological framework of hippocampal dysfunction in aging and disease. Nature Reviews Neuroscience, 12(10), 585-601.

Smith, A. D., & Refsum, H. (2016). Homocysteine, B Vitamins, and cognitive impairment. Annual review of nutrition, 36, 211-239.

Smith, A. D., Refsum, H., Bottiglieri, T., Fenech, M., Hooshmand, B., Mccaddon, A.,... Obeid, R. (2018). Homocysteine and Dementia: An International Consensus Statement1. Journal of Alzheimer's Disease,62(2), 561- 570.

Spira, A. P., Gamaldo, A. A., An, Y., Wu, M. N., Simonsick, E. M., Bilgel, M., ... & Resnick, S. M. (2013). Self-reported sleep and β-amyloid deposition in community-dwelling older adults. Jama neurology, 70(12), 1537-1543.

Stanford Health Care. (2019, August 21). How is dementia diagnosed?

Stanford Health Care. (2017, September 11). Psychiatric Evaluation.

Stern, Y., Albert, S., Tang, M. X., & Tsai, W. Y. (1999). Rate of memory decline in AD is related to education and occupation: cognitive reserve? Neurology, 53(9), 1942-1942.

Stroop, J. R. (1935). Studies of interference in serial verbal reactions. Journal of experimental psychology, 18(6), 643.

Teixeira, C. V. L., Guedes, R. V. S., Ribeiro, N. F., & Pereira, A. (2013). Effect of Indian gooseberry (Emblica officinalis) on plasma antioxidant potential and skin characteristics in aged mice: a preliminary study. Pharmaceutical biology, 51(9), 1174-1178.

Thomas, A. J., Ferrier, I. N., Kalaria, R. N., Davis, S., O'Brien, J. T., Ballard, C., & Perry, R. (2001). Elevation in late-life depression of intercellular adhesion molecule-1 expression in the dorsolateral prefrontal cortex. The American journal of psychiatry, 158(11), 1872-1878.

Tomlinson, B. E., Blessed, G., & Roth, M. (1970). Observations on the brains of demented old people. Journal of the Neurological Sciences, 11(3), 205-242.

Tsai, J., Grutzendler, J., Duff, K., & Gan, W. B. (2004). Fibrillar amyloid deposition leads to local synaptic abnormalities and breakage of neuronal branches. Nature Neuroscience, 7(11), 1181-1183.

U.S. National Library of Medicine - MedlinePlus. (2020, June 17). Dementia.

Van der Flier, W. M., & Scheltens, P. (2005). Epidemiology and risk factors of dementia. Journal of Neurology, Neurosurgery, and Psychiatry, 76(Suppl 5), v2-v7.

Wagner U, Echterhoff G. When Does Oxytocin Affect Human Memory Encoding? The Role of Social Context and Individual Attachment Style. Front Hum Neurosci. 2018 Sep 20; 12:349. doi: 10.3389/fnhum.2018.00349. PMID: 30294265; PMCID: PMC6158322

Yang, H. D., Kim, D. H., Lee, S. B., & Young, L. D. (2016). History of Alzheimer's Disease. Dementia and Neurocognitive Disorders, 15(4), 121.

Yesavage, J. A., Brink, T. L., Rose, T. L., Lum, O., Huang, V., Adey, M., & Leirer, V. O. (1983). Development and validation of a geriatric depression scale: a preliminary report. Journal of psychiatric research, 17(1), 37-49.

Yoon, C. W., Shin, J. S., Kim, H. J., Cho, H., Noh, Y., Kim, G. H., ... & Kim, C. (2014). Cognitive deficits of pure subcortical vascular dementia vs. Alzheimer disease: PiB-PET-based study. Neurology, 82(7), 569-573.

Zhou, J., Peng, W., Xu, M., Li, W., & Liu, Z. (2015). The Effectiveness and Safety of Acupuncture for Patients with Alzheimer's Disease. Medicine, 94(22).

Zlokovic, B. V. (2011). Neurovascular pathways to neurodegeneration in Alzheimer's disease and other disorders. Nature Reviews Neuroscience, 12(12), 723-738.

www.ingramcontent.com/pod-product-compliance
Lightning Source LLC
Chambersburg PA
CBHW070752270326
41927CB00010B/2115